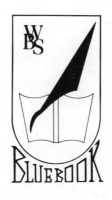

BLUEBOOK

ON CALL

principles and protocols

Jean H. Gillies, M.D., F.R.C.P.C.

Department of Medicine
St. Paul's Hospital
University of British Columbia
Vancouver, British Columbia, Canada

Shane A. Marshall, M.D., F.R.C.P.C.

Department of Medicine
St. Paul's Hospital
University of British Columbia
Vancouver, British Columbia, Canada

John Ruedy, M.D., F.R.C.P.C.

Head, Department of Medicine
St. Paul's Hospital
University of British Columbia
Vancouver, British Columbia, Canada

1989
W.B. SAUNDERS COMPANY
Harcourt Brace Jovanovich, Inc.

Philadelphia   London   Toronto
Montreal   Sydney   Tokyo

W. B. SAUNDERS COMPANY
Harcourt Brace Jovanovich, Inc.

The Curtis Center
Independence Square West
Philadelphia, PA 19106

Library of Congress Cataloging-in-Publication Data

Gillies, Jean H.
  On call.

  Includes index.

1. Medical emergencies.   2. Hospitals—Medical staff.
  I. Marshall, Shane A.   II. Ruedy, John.   III. Title.

RC86.7.G55 1989   616'.025   88-18306

ISBN 0-7216-2576-2

Editor: John Dyson
Developmental Editor: David Kilmer
Designer: Patti Maddaloni
Production Manager: Pete Faber
Manuscript Editor: Mary Anne Folcher
Illustration Coordinator: Brett MacNaughton
Indexer: Dorothy Stade

On Call: Principles and Protocols   ISBN 0–7216–2576–2

Last digit is the print number: 9   8   7   6   5   4   3   2

INTRODUCTORY NOTE

Each volume in the Saunders Blue Books® Series is intended to be a practical aid for primary care physicians, house officers, and medical students in clinical training. Each Blue Book presents the latest diagnostic and therapeutic information pertinent to its clinical field. Above all else, these books are intended to be useful in the real world of providing daily patient care. Their convenient format allows maximal retrieval of relevant information in a minimum of time.

Our Series derives its name from the "Blue Series"—the first books published by the W.B. Saunders Company 100 years ago. That Series, like its modern descendant, was intended to sort out important scientific and clinical facts that would aid the physician or the student in training. Today, as medical information grows exponentially, health professionals recognize their obligation both to remain current and to select from the engulfing sea of clinical data those particular pieces that will aid them in their practice. The volumes in Saunders Blue Books® Series will help them achieve these goals. They should be regarded as portable clinical tools—useful, always on call, and ready to help when needed.

MICKEY S. EISENBERG, M.D., PH.D.
Consulting Editor

To our families in
Bermuda, Canada, and England.

PREFACE

The responsibility for calls at night is one of the traditional duties of medical students and residents in teaching hospitals. *On Call: Principles and Protocols* is designed to facilitate the transition of medical students and residents from the classroom to the hospital setting. We believe that the initiation of the medical student to hospital practice need not be one of trial and error and need not be recalled as a year of stress and uncertainty.

On Call emphasizes the assessment and management of the common problems for which medical students and residents are called at night. The approach of the book is unique in providing both instruction and reference, while emphasizing the rational thought processes required for optimal patient care in specific clinical situations. It is our belief that this structured approach deserves greater emphasis in the undergraduate years, and we are hopeful that it will help in the introduction of students to clinical medicine.

JEAN GILLIES
SHANE MARSHALL
JOHN RUEDY

ACKNOWLEDGEMENTS

We are grateful to the many reviewers of this text from St. Paul's Hospital who provided helpful and detailed comments on individual chapters: Drs. A. Anzarut, C. Chan-Yan, S. Clarke, R. Conn, A. Dodek, J. Kennedy, D. Landsberg, L. Lawson, I. MacDonald, W. A. McLeod, J. McCormack, J. Onrot, T. Phang, L. Rabeneck, J. Russell, C. Thompson, H. Tildesley, L. Vickars, R. Werb, and P. Wilcox. We would also like to extend thanks to Dr. Andy Pattullo for his excellent contributions to the illustrations in the text; to Mrs. Dickie Bruce for her unfailing patience, sense of humor, and excellent secretarial assistance; and to Miss Debbie Spring for her hours and hours of typing.

DOSAGE NOTICE

Extraordinary efforts have been made by the authors, the editors, and the publisher of this book to ensure that dosage recommendations are precise and in agreement with the highest standards of practice. [The drug dosage recommendations are those for adults.]

Dosage schedules are changed from time to time in the light of accumulating clinical experience and continuing laboratory studies. These changes are most likely to occur in the case of recently introduced products.

We urge, therefore, that you check the package information data for the manufacturer's recommended dosage. In addition, there are some quite serious situations, each encountered only rarely, in which drug therapy must be individualized, and expert judgment advises the use of a higher dosage or administration by a different route than is included in the manufacturer's recommendations.

STRUCTURE OF THE BOOK

The book is divided into three sections.

Section I covers introductory material in three separate chapters: (1) Approach to the Diagnosis and Management of On-Call Problems, (2) Documentation of On-Call Problems, and (3) Assessment and Management of Volume Status. Volume status is discussed in the introductory section as its assessment is essential in the proper management of almost all problems in hospitalized patients.

Section II contains the 20 common calls associated with patient-related problems. Each problem is approached from its inception, beginning with the relevant questions that should be asked over the phone, the temporary orders that should be given, and the major life-threatening problems to be considered as one approaches the bedside.

- PHONE CALLS
  Questions—pertinent questions in order to assess the urgency of the situation.
  Orders—urgent orders to be carried out before the housestaff arrives at the bedside.
  Inform the RN—RN to be informed of the time the housestaff anticipates arrival at the bedside.
- ELEVATOR THOUGHTS
  The differential diagnosis to be considered by the housestaff while they are on their way to assess the patient (i.e., while they are in the elevator).
- MAJOR THREAT TO LIFE
  Identification of the major threat to life is essential in providing focus for the subsequent effective management of the patient.
- BEDSIDE
  The quick-look test is a rapid visual assessment to place the patient into one of three categories: well, sick, or critical. This helps determine the necessity of immediate intervention.
  Vital Signs
  Selective history
  Selective physical examination
  Management

Section III contains the five common calls associated with laboratory-related problems.

The Appendices consist of reference items that we have found useful in managing calls.

COMMONLY USED ABBREVIATIONS

ABD	Abdomen
ABG	Arterial blood gas
AC	Before meals
ACTH	Adrenocorticotropic hormone
AIDS	Acquired immune deficiency syndrome
ANA	Antinuclear antibody
A/P	Anteroposterior
aPTT	Activated partial thromboplastin time
ARDS	Adult respiratory distress syndrome
ASD	Atrial septal defect
AV	Atrioventricular
BP	Blood pressure
BPH	Benign prostatic hypertrophy
CBC	Complete blood count
CCU	Coronary care unit
CGL	Chronic granulocytic leukemia
CHF	Congestive heart failure
CLL	Chronic lymphocytic leukemia
CMV	Cytomegalovirus
CNS	Central nervous system
CO	Cardiac output
COPD	Chronic obstructive pulmonary disease
CPK	Creatine phosphokinase
CrCl	Creatinine clearance
C+S	Culture and sensitivity
CT	Computerized tomography
CVS	Cardiovascular system
CXR	Chest X-ray
D5W	5% dextrose in water
DDAVP	1-desamino-(8-D-arginine)-vasopressin
DIC	Disseminated intravascular coagulation
D5NS	5% dextrose in normal saline
DVT	Deep venous thrombosis
ECF	Extracellular fluid
ECG	Electrocardiogram
EDTA	Disodium edetate
ENDO	Endocrine
ENT	Ears, nose, and throat
ESR	Erythrocyte sedimentation rate
EXT	Extremities
FDP	Fibrin degradation products

FIO_2	Fraction of inspired oxygen
FUO	Fever of unknown origin
GI	Gastrointestinal
G-6-PD	Glucose-6-phosphate dehydrogenase
GTT	Glucose tolerance test
GU	Genitourinary
Hb	Hemoglobin
HEENT	Head, eyes, ears, nose, and throat
HIV	Human immunodeficiency virus
HJR	Hepatojugular reflux
HPI	History of present illness
hs	Hora somni (at bedtime)
HR	Heart rate
IBW	Ideal body weight
ICF	Intracellular fluid
ICU	Intensive care unit
ICU/CCU	Intensive care unit/coronary care unit
IDDM	Insulin-dependent diabetes mellitus
IM	Intramuscular
ITP	Idiopathic thrombocytopenic purpura
IV	Intravenous
IVAC	Infusion pump
IVP	Intravenous pyelogram
J	Joule's equivalent
JVP	Jugular venous pressure
L	Liter
LDH	Lactate dehydrogenase
LLQ	Lower left quadrant
LOC	Level of consciousness
LP	Lumbar puncture
LUQ	Left upper quadrant
MAO	Monoamine oxidase
MCV	Mean corpuscular volume
MD	Doctor of medicine
MI	Myocardial infarction
MISC	Miscellaneous
MSS	Musculoskeletal system
MVP	Mitral valve prolapse
NEURO	Neurological system
NG	Nasogastric
NIDDM	Non-insulin dependent diabetes mellitus
NPH	Neutral protamine Hagedorn (Insulin)
NPO	Nil per os (nothing by mouth)
NS	Normal saline (0.9% saline in water)
NSAID	Nonsteroidal anti-inflammatory drug
NYD	Not yet diagnosed
P/A	Posteroanterior
PAC	Premature atrial contraction

PAT	Paroxysmal atrial tachycardia
PC	After meals
P_{CO_2}	Partial pressure of carbon dioxide
PMNs	Polymorphonuclear cells
PND	Paroxysmal nocturnal dyspnea
PO	Per os (by mouth)
P_{O_2}	Partial pressure of oxygen
PR	Per rectum
PRN	As necessary
PT	Prothrombin time
PTT	Partial thromboplastin time
PUD	Peptic ulcer disease
PVC	Premature ventricular contraction
QID	Four times a day
R1	Resident
RA	Rheumatoid arthritis
RAD	Right axis deviation
RBBB	Right bundle branch block
RBC	Red blood cell
RESP	Respiratory system
RLQ	Right lower quadrant
RN	Registered nurse
ROM	Range of motion
RR	Respiratory rate
RTA	Renal tubular acidosis
RUQ	Right upper quadrant
RV	Right ventricle
S_3	Third heart sound
SAH	Subarachnoid hemorrhage
SBE	Subacute bacterial endocarditis (infectious endocarditis)
SC	Subcutaneous
SI	International System of Units
SIADH	Syndrome of inappropriate antidiuretic hormone
SL	Sublingual
SLE	Systemic lupus erythematosis
SOB	Shortness of breath
SSS	Sick sinus syndrome
stat	Immediately
STS	Serologic test for syphilis
SVT	Supraventricular tachycardia
T_4	Thyroxine
TB	Tuberculosis
TBW	Total body water
TIA	Transient ischemic attack
TKVO	To keep vein open
TPN	Total parenteral nutrition
TSH	Thyroid stimulating hormone

TTP	Thrombotic thrombocytopenic purpura
URTI	Upper respiratory tract infection
UTI	Urinary tract infection
VP	Ventriculoperitoneal
VSD	Ventricular septal defect
WBC	White blood count
ZN	Ziehl-Neelsen

CONTENTS

INTRODUCTION TO DIAGNOSIS, MANAGEMENT, DOCUMENTATION, AND VOLUME STATUS

PATIENT-RELATED PROBLEMS: THE 20 COMMON CALLS

LABORATORY-RELATED PROBLEMS: THE FIVE COMMON CALLS

INTRODUCTION TO DIAGNOSIS, MANAGEMENT, DOCUMENTATION AND VOLUME STATUS

1

APPROACH TO THE DIAGNOSIS AND MANAGEMENT OF ON-CALL PROBLEMS

Clinical problem solving is an important function required by the physician on-call. Historically, a physician approaches the diagnosis and management of a patient's problems with an ordered, structured system (e.g., history-taking, physical examination, review of available tests, and x-rays) prior to the formulation of the provisional and differential diagnoses and the management plan. The history-taking and physical examination may take 30 to 40 minutes for an otherwise well patient presenting with a single problem to the family physician for the first time, or they may take 60 to 90 minutes for a geriatric patient presenting with multiple complaints. Clearly, if the patient presents to the emergency room unconscious, having been found on the street, then the chief complaint is coma, and the HPI is limited to the minimal information provided by the ambulance attendants or by the contents of the patient's wallet. In this situation, physicians are trained to proceed with examination, investigation, and treatment "concurrently." How this is to be achieved is not always clear, although there is agreement on the steps that should be completed within the initial 5 to 10 minutes.

The physician is first confronted with on-call problem solving in the final years of medical school. It is at this stage that the structured history-taking and physical examination system directs the student's approach in evaluating a patient. The medical student is faced with well-defined problems when on-call (e.g., fall-out-of-bed, fever, chest pain) yet feels ill equipped to begin clinical problem solving unless it involves "the complete history and physical." Anything less than the 60 minutes (usually more) "admission history and physical" engenders guilt over a task only partially completed, yet every on-call problem cannot involve 60 minutes or more of the physician's time, since inadequate treatment time will be given to sick patients because of the unnecessary time spent on relatively minor problems.

The approach recommended in this book offers a structured system, but one that can be logically adapted to most situations. It is intended as a practical guide to assist in efficient clinical problem solving when on-call. Chapters so related are divided into four parts as follows:
1. Phone call
2. Elevator thoughts
3. Major threat to life
4. Bedside

PHONE CALL

Most problems confronting the physician on-call are first communicated by telephone. The physician must be able to determine the severity of the problem over the telephone, since it is not always possible to immediately assess the patient at the bedside. Patients must be evaluated in order of priority. The phone call section of each chapter is divided into three parts as follows:

1. Questions
2. Orders
3. Inform RN

The questions are selected to assist in determining the urgency of the problem. Orders are suggested that will help expedite the investigation and management of urgent situations. Finally, the RN is informed of the physician's anticipated time of arrival at the bedside, and the responsibilities of the RN in the interim.

ELEVATOR THOUGHTS

Since the physician on-call is not usually on the floor when he or she is informed of a problem that requires assessment, the time spent travelling to the ward, which may be up to 10 minutes in some large hospital complexes, may be used efficiently to consider the differential diagnosis of the problem at hand. Since time is spent standing still in the elevator, the term "elevator thoughts" has been coined to summarize the directed differential diagnosis. It should be emphasized that the differential diagnosis lists that are offered are not exhaustive but rather focus on the most common or the most serious (life-threatening) causes that should be considered in hospitalized patients.

MAJOR THREAT TO LIFE

Identification of the major threat to life that each problem presents provides a focus for the subsequent effective investigation and management of the patient. The major threat to life posed by each problem follows logically from a consideration of the differential diagnosis. Rather than arriving at the bedside with a memorized list of possible diagnoses, an appreciation of the one or two most likely threats to life is more useful and relevant in directing one's questions and physical examination. This mental process serves to ensure that the most serious life-threatening possibility in each clinical scenario is both considered and sought after in the initial evaluation of the patient.

BEDSIDE

The protocols for what to do upon arrival at the bedside are divided into the following parts:

- Quick look test
- Airway and vital signs
- Selective history
- Selective physical examination
- Selective chart review
- Management

The bedside assessment should begin with the "quick look test" and "airway and vital signs." The quick look test is a rapid visual assessment that may enable the physician to categorize the patient's condition into one of three degrees of severity; well (comfortable), sick (uncomfortable or distressed), or critical (about to die). Next is assessment of the airway and the vital signs, important in the evaluation of any potentially sick patient. Because of the nature of the various problems that require assessment when on-call, the order of the remaining parts is not uniform. For example, in Chapter 4 *Abdominal Pain* follows the expected sequence of Selective History and Chart Review, Selective Physical Examination and Management, whereas in Chapter 19 *Seizures* follows the sequence of Management I, Selective Physical Examination I, Selective History and Chart Review, Selective Physical Examination II, and Management II. Occasionally, Selective Physical Examination and Management sections are subdivided. This division allows for the first focus on the urgent, life-threatening problem, leaving the less urgent problems to be reviewed in the second subdivision.

It is hoped that the principles and protocols offered for clinical problem solving of common on-call problems will provide a logical, efficient system for the assessment and management of patients in the hospital.

2

DOCUMENTATION OF ON-CALL PROBLEMS

Accurate, concise documentation of on-call problems at night is essential for the continued efficient care of hospitalized patients. In many instances the patient you are asked to see at night will not be known to you, and you may not be involved in their continuing care after your night on-call. Some problems can safely be handled over the telephone, but in the majority of situations a selective history and physical examination will be required in order to correctly diagnose and treat the problem. Documentation is recommended on every patient you examine; if the problem is straightforward your note can be brief, and if the problem is complicated, your note should be concise yet complete.

Begin by recording the date, time, and who you are, e.g., Aug 10, 1987 0200H. "Medical student on-call note" or "Intern on-call note."
State who called you and at what time you were called, e.g., Called to see patient by RN at 0130H because the patient "fell-out-of-bed."

If your assessment is delayed by more urgent problems, say so. A brief one or two sentence summary of the patient's admission diagnosis and major medical problems should follow:

This 74-year-old woman, with a history of chronic renal failure, NIDDM, and rheumatoid arthritis was admitted 10 days ago with increasing joint pain.

Next describe the HPI of the "fall-out-of-bed" both from the patient's viewpoint and from that of any witnesses. The HPI is no different from the HPI you would document in your admission history, e.g.:

HPI. The patient was on the way to the bathroom to void, tripped on her bathrobe, and fell to the floor, landing on her left side. She denied palpitations, chest pain, lightheadedness, nausea, and hip pain. There was no difficulty walking unaided and no pain afterwards. The fall was not witnessed; the RN found the patient lying on the floor. Vital signs were stable.

If your chart review has relevant findings, include these in your HPI, e.g.:

Three previous "falls-out-of-bed" on this admission—patient has no recall of these events.

Documentation of your examination should be selective; a call regarding a fall-out-of-bed requires you to examine relevant components of the vital signs, head and neck, cardiovascular, musculoskeletal, and neurologic systems.

It is not necessary to examine the respiratory system or the abdomen, unless there is a second separate problem (e.g., you arrive at the bedside and find the patient febrile). On-call problems should not require you to take a complete history and conduct a complete physical examination; these have already been done when the patient was admitted. Your history, physical examination, and chart documentation should be directed (i.e., problem oriented). It may be useful to underline the positive physical findings both for yourself (it aids your summary) and for the housestaff who will be following the patient in the morning as follows:

PHYSICAL EXAMINATION

VITALS	BP 140/85
	HR <u>104</u> beats/min
	RR <u>36</u> min
	Temp <u>38.9</u> PO
HEENT	No tongue or cheek lacerations
	No hemotympanum
CVS	Pulse rate and rhythm normal; JVP 2 cm > SA
MSS	No skull or face lacerations or hematomas
	Spine and ribs normal
	Full, painless ROM of all 4 limbs normal
	Reflexes ⎫
	Motor ⎬ Normal
	Sensory ⎭
NEURO	Alert. Oriented to time, place, and person.

Relevant laboratory, ECG, or x-ray findings should be documented. Again it is useful to underline abnormal findings, e.g.,

- Glucose   7.2 mmol/L
- Sodium   141 mmol/L
- Potassium 3.9 mmol/L
- Calcium   not available
- Urea   <u>12 mmol/L</u>
- Creatinine <u>180 mmol/L</u>

Your diagnostic conclusion, regarding the problem for which you were called, must be clearly stated. It is not enough to write "patient fell-out-of-bed"—the RN could have written that without ever seeing the patient. The information gathered must be synthesized to achieve the highest level of diagnostic integration plausible. This "provisional diagnosis" should be followed by a differential diagnosis in order of the most likely alternative explanations. In the patient who "fell-out-of-bed," your diagnostic conclusion might be as follows:

1. "Fall-out-of-bed" due to difficulty reaching the bathroom to void (? diuretic-induced nocturia, ? contribution of hs sedation).
2. Large hematoma (7 × 9 cm) left thigh.

Your "plan" must be clearly stated, both the measures taken during the night and the investigations or treatment you have organized for the morning. Avoid writing "Plan—see orders": it is not always obvious to the staff taking over the next day why certain measures were taken. If you informed the intern, resident, or attending physician of the problem, document with whom you spoke and the recommendations given. Record whether any of the patient's family members were informed of the problem and what they were told. Lastly, sign or print your name clearly so the staff know who to contact should they have any questions regarding the management of this patient the following day.

3

ASSESSMENT AND MANAGEMENT OF VOLUME STATUS

The assessment of volume status is an integral part of the physical examination. You will find in your years as a medical student and intern and later as a practicing physician that this skill plays a key role in helping to choose the appropriate investigation and management in many clinical situations.

Ideally, this skill is best learned at the bedside. However, some background knowledge will help you in the accurate assessment and interpretation of a patient's volume status.

First, terminology must be clarified. The human body is composed mostly of water (Fig. 3–1). In fact, *total body water* (TBW) makes up 60% of the weight of the adult male. Of this, 75% is made up of *intracellular fluid* (ICF), and 25% is made up of *extracellular fluid* (ECF), i.e., water that is "outside" of cells. Of the extracellular fluid, 66% is made up of *interstitial fluid,* such as fluid bathing the cells, cerebrospinal fluid, and intraocular fluid. Only 5% of total body water consists of *intravascular fluid* (plasma).

Clinically, it is the extracellular fluid, consisting of intravascular and interstitial fluids, that one is trying to assess when determining the volume status of a patient.

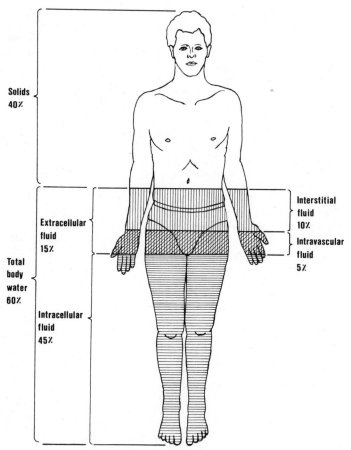

Figure 3–1. Body fluid compartments.

THE ASSESSMENT OF VOLUME STATUS

There are only three basic states of volume status that a patient can have—volume depleted, normovolemic ("euvolemic"), and volume overloaded. On approaching the bedside, ask yourself whether the patient is volume depleted, normovolemic, or volume overloaded.

QUICK LOOK TEST

Does the patient look well (comfortable), sick (uncomfortable or distressed), or critical (about to die)?
In most instances as you enter the patient's room and first see the patient, it will become apparent whether there is a serious fluid balance abnormality. Most patients who look well are normovolemic, whereas patients who look sick are seriously volume depleted or volume overloaded. Of course, this is a general guideline only, and a more detailed physical examination is required.

VITAL SIGNS

In most cases, simply taking the patient's vital signs will help you determine whether or not there is significant volume depletion.
Measure the heart rate and blood pressure first with the patient supine and then after the patient stands for 1 minute. If the patient is unable to stand alone ask for assistance from the nursing or orderly staff. If the patient is hypotensive in the supine position, this maneuver is not necessary.

An increase in heart rate > 15 beats/min, a fall in systolic blood pressure > 15 mm Hg, or any fall in diastolic blood pressure indicates significant *intravascular volume depletion.*

A patient with autonomic dysfunction (e.g., beta blockers, diabetic neuropathy, Shy-Drager syndrome) may also have a pronounced postural fall in BP but without the expected degree of compensatory tachycardia. Unlike the volume depleted patient, however, there should be no other features of extracellular fluid deficit in the patient with uncomplicated autonomic dysfunction.

A resting tachycardia may be seen with either volume depletion or volume overload. *Volume depletion* results in a low stroke volume, as can be seen from the following formula, and hence the patient must generate a tachycardia in order to maintain cardiac output.

$$\text{Cardiac Output} = \text{Heart Rate} \times \text{Stroke Volume}$$
$$(\text{CO}) = (\text{HR}) \times (\text{SV})$$

The volume overloaded patient must also generate a tachycardia in an effort to increase forward flow and thereby relieve the lungs of hypoxia-causing pulmonary congestion. A *normovolemic* patient without other complicating features will have a normal heart rate.

Measure the respiratory rate. The most important feature to look for when measuring the respiratory rate is tachypnea, which may be seen in the volume overloaded patient in whom pulmonary edema has developed.

SELECTIVE PHYSICAL EXAMINATION

HEENT   *Look at the oral mucous membranes.* The adequately hydrated patient has moist mucous membranes. It is normal for a small "pool" of saliva to collect at the undersurface of the tongue in the area of the frenulum, and this should be looked for.

RESP   *Listen for crackles.* Pulmonary edema with bilateral basilar crackles and, occasionally, wheezes or pleural effusions may be a manifestation of the volume over-loaded patient.

CVS   *Look at the neck veins.* Examination of the internal jugular veins is one of the most helpful components of the volume status examination. The JVP may be assessed with the patient at any inclination from 0 degrees to 90 degrees. However, it is easiest to begin looking for the JVP pulsation with the patient at a 45 degree inclination. If, at 45 degrees, you are unable to visualize the neck veins, then this usually signifies that the JVP is either very low (in which case you will need to lower the head of the bed) or very high (in which case you may need to sit the patient upright in order to see the top of the column of blood in the internal jugular vein). Once the internal jugular vein pulsation is identified, measure the perpendicular distance from the sternal angle to the top of the column of blood (Fig. 3–2). This distance represents the patient's JVP in cm H_2O above the sternal angle.

A JVP of 2 to 3 cm above the sternal angle is normal in the adult patient. A significantly *volume depleted* patient will have flat neck veins, which may fill only when the patient is placed in Trendelenburg's position. A *volume overloaded* patient will usually have an elevated JVP greater than 3 cm above the sternal angle.

Listen for an S_3. An S_3 is most often associated with the volume overloaded state and, sometimes, may be heard only in the left lateral position.

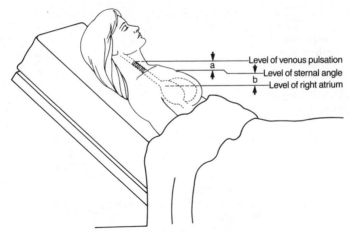

Figure 3–2. Measurement of jugular venous pressure. a = The perpendicular distance from the sternal angle to the top of the column of blood and b = the distance from the center of the right atrium to the sternal angle, commonly accepted as measuring 5 cm, regardless of inclination.

ABD   *Examine the liver.* An enlarged, tender liver and a positive hepatojugular reflux may be manifestations of the volume overloaded state.

SKIN   *Check the skin turgor.* Evaluating the skin turgor in an adult is best performed by raising a fold of skin from the anterior chest area over the sternal angle. In an adequately hydrated patient the skin should promptly return to its usual position. This is a useful test for identifying *interstitial fluid deficits.*

Look at the skin creases and check for edema. Accentuated skin creases from bed sheets' pressing against the posterior thorax and sacral or pedal edema indicate *interstitial fluid excess.*

SELECTIVE CHART REVIEW

Sometimes it is difficult to decide at the bedside whether or not a patient's volume status is normal. There are then a few things in the chart that may help guide you in a difficult case.

Look at the Creatinine/Urea Ratio. A ratio of less than 12 (calculated in SI units) is suggestive of volume depletion.

Examine the Fluid Balance Records. Unfortunately, fluid balance records are often notoriously inaccurate. However, if well-kept records are present, a number of clues may be found. A patient who is taking in very little fluid (whether orally or intravenously) may well be volume depleted. A patient whose urine output is greater than 20 ml/hr is probably not volume depleted. A net positive intake of several liters over a few days may be indicative of fluid retention with concomitant volume overload.

In the Volume Depleted Patient, Look at the Chart for Contributing Causes

GI Losses	Vomiting
	Nasogastric suction
	Diarrhea
Urinary Losses	Diuretics
	Osmotic diuresis (hyperglycemia, mannitol administration, hypertonic IV contrast material)
	Diabetes insipidus
	Recovery phase of acute tubular necrosis
	Adrenal insufficiency
Surface Losses	Skin (increased sweating due to fever, evaporation in burn patients)
	Respiratory tract (hyperventilation, non-humidified inhalation therapy)
Fluid Sequestration	Pancreatitis
	Ileus
	Burns
Blood Losses	GI tract
	Surgical
	Iatrogenic (laboratory sampling)
Other	Inadequate oral or parenteral intake

It is a rare occasion when a patient has every feature of volume depletion or volume overload. Still, it is useful when examining a patient to carry a mental picture of the three "classic" states of volume status.

The Classic Volume Depleted Patient

Quick Look Test
The patient looks sick.

Vital Signs
HR	Resting tachycardia
	Postural rise in HR > 15 beats/min
BP	Normal or low resting BP
	A postural drop in systolic BP > 15 mm Hg or any drop in diastolic BP
RR	Normal

HEENT	Dry oral mucous membranes
RESP	Clear
CVS	JVP flat
	No S_3
ABD	Normal
SKIN	Poor turgor
	No edema

The Classic Volume Overloaded Patient

Quick Look Test

The patient looks sick and short of breath. Often he or she will be sitting upright.

Vital Signs

HR	Resting tachycardia
	Postural rise in HR < 15 beats/min
BP	May be low, normal, or high
	No postural fall in systolic or diastolic BP
RR	Tachypnea
RESP	Crackles bilaterally at bases
	± Wheezing
	± Pleural effusions
CVS	JVP > 3 cm above the sternal angle
	S_3 present
ABD	Positive hepatojugular reflux
	± Enlarged tender liver
EXT	Accentuated skin folds on posterior thorax
	Sacral or pedal edema

The Classic Patient with a Normal Volume Status

Quick Look Test

The patient looks well.

Vital Signs

HR	Normal
	Postural rise in HR < 15 beats/min
BP	Normal
	Postural fall of systolic BP < 15 mm Hg and no fall in diastolic BP
RR	Normal
HEENT	Moist oral mucous membranes
RESP	Clear
CVS	JVP 2 to 3 cm above the sternal angle
	No S_3
ABD	Normal
EXT	No edema

CHOOSING THE CORRECT INTRAVENOUS FLUID

Selection of an appropriate intravenous fluid for a particular clinical situation need not be a guessing game. A basic understanding of physiology will help to make your fluid management decisions rational and effective.

Water is important in the body because it serves as a *solvent* for a variety of solutes. *Solutes* can be either electrolytes or non-electrolytes. If you read any patient's chart and turn to the laboratory section, you will see a number of electrolytes and non-electrolytes that can be measured.

Electrolytes are substances in which the molecules dissociate into charged components (ions) when placed in water, and they include the following commonly measured substances:

- Sodium ⎫
- Potassium ⎬ cations
- Calcium ⎪
- Magnesium ⎭

- Chloride ⎫
- Bicarbonate ⎬ anions

In physiologic solutions the total number of cations always equals the total number of anions.

Non-electrolytes are solutes that have no electrical charges, and they include such substances as glucose and urea.

As mentioned previously, most blood volume is made up of *water,* which acts as a solvent to dissolve and transport electrolytes and non-electrolytes. Water is able to move from one body compartment to the next by the process of *osmosis.* When two solutes are separated by a semi-permeable membrane, such as a cell membrane, water will tend to flow across the membrane from the solution of lower concentration to that of higher concentration, the net effect being to equalize the solute concentration on each side of the membrane (Fig. 3–3).

Suppose you were seeing a patient in whom you had decided to infuse a liter of pure water without any solutes. What would happen to the patient's red blood cells? Understanding the process of osmosis allows you to reason that since the solute concentration inside the red blood cells is vastly higher than that in the water infused, water would move across the cell membrane into the red blood cells (Fig. 3–4). There is a limit to how much the red blood cell membrane can stretch, and eventually the red blood cells would burst.

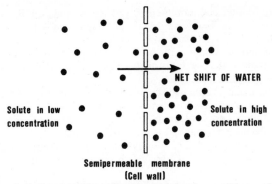

NET SHIFT OF WATER

Solute in low
concentration

Solute in high
concentration

Semipermeable membrane
(Cell wall)

Figure 3–3. Osmosis. Water flows across a semipermeable membrane in order to equalize solute concentrations on either side of the membrane.

Similarly, you can see that if a hypertonic solution was infused directly into the patient's vein, the red blood cells would shrink (crenate), as water moved out of the red blood cells and into the surrounding solution.

For these reasons, most intravenous fluids that are prepared for hospital use are usually close to isotonic, i.e., they have the same solute concentration as the blood to minimize such fluid shifts.

Although cell membranes allow water to pass freely by the process of osmosis, such membranes fortunately limit the passage of solutes to a varying degree. Some solute molecules cross membranes more readily than others, depending on their size and physical properties.

In the hospitalized patient there are only three solutes that you need to know about in order to effectively diagnose and treat disorders of fluid balance. Glucose distributes widely throughout both intracellular and extracellular spaces, whereas sodium is limited to the extracellular space. Albumin remains largely within the intravascular space. The distribution that these three solutes have is a fundamental principle that you will find useful in guiding your decisions regarding choice of fluid therapy.

D5W consists of 50 gm of dextrose dissolved in a liter of water. It has an osmolality of 252 mOsm/L, which will prevent the patient's red blood cells from shrinking or swelling. D5W can be expected to equilibrate rapidly among the intravascular, extracellular, and intracellular spaces, and water will follow along quickly by osmosis.

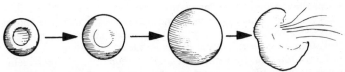

Figure 3–4. Osmosis. Effect of infusion of pure water on RBC volume.

NS is another commonly employed intravenous solution. It has an osmolality of 308 mOsm/L and, although slightly hypertonic, is not different enough from blood tonicity to cause cell shrinkage. NS will stay predominantly in the extracellular space somewhat longer than a glucose infusion because sodium does not readily move intracellularly.

Albumin and *plasma* will stay in the intravascular space for many hours since albumin is a large molecule that does not easily traverse the endothelial pores of the blood vessels. The half-life of albumin within the intravascular space is 17 to 20 hours.

From this knowledge of solutes and their membrane permeability, it will be easy to make logical choices regarding fluid management.

In patients with *extravascular volume depletion* the goal of treatment is to correct and maintain adequate intravascular volume and tissue perfusion. Hence, the volume depleted patient could be treated with intravenous NS, albumin, or plasma. Because NS is more readily available and much less expensive, it is the treatment of choice for the initial resuscitation of the volume depleted patient. Infusing D5W would be of little benefit since the glucose and water would distribute throughout the intravascular and extravascular spaces.

In patients with *extravascular volume excess* the goal of treatment is to improve and maintain adequate cardiac function and tissue perfusion. These usually require the use of preload reducing measures, as outlined in Chapter 20, page 206. However, because these patients are often critically ill, they require intravenous access for medication administration. The best choice of fluid to give, usually at a TKVO rate, is D5W which will very quickly leave the intravascular space. Infusing NS or albumin could worsen the patient's condition by further increasing intravascular volume. This is why cardiac patients, who are at risk for volume overload, are usually given an IV of D5W when IV access is required for administration of medication.

Another IV solution, "2/3rds 1/3rd," contains 33 gm/L of glucose and 51 mmol/L each of sodium and chloride and is approximately isotonic at 269 mOsm/L. Although there is no particular physiologic basis for its use, it has been popularized as a "maintenance IV solution" for patients in whom adequate oral intake cannot be met.

Remember. Correct volume status abnormalities at a rate similar to the rate at which they developed. Biologic systems are more responsive to rates of change than to absolute amounts of change. It is safest to correct half the deficit and then re-evaluate. There is no substitute for frequent repeated examination of the patient when trying to effect changes in volume status.

Occasionally, you will be faced with a patient in whom there is

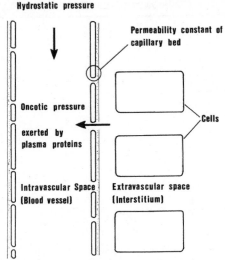

Figure 3–5. Factors influencing fluid transfer between the intravascular and extravascular spaces.

a discrepancy between the two compartments of the extracellular fluid, e.g., the patient with a decreased intravascular volume but an excess of interstitial fluid (i.e., edema). This discrepancy is most commonly seen in states of marked hypoalbuminemia.

Fluid transfer from the intravascular space to the extravascular space (interstitium) depends on the permeability of the capillary bed, how much hydrostatic pressure is being exerted to force fluid out of the intravascular space, and the difference in *oncotic pressure* between the intravascular and extravascular spaces (Fig. 3–5).

Oncotic pressure is exerted by *plasma protein* (i.e., albumin). There is little, if any, protein in the interstitium, and hence the intravascular oncotic pressure exerted by albumin tends to draw water out of the interstitium and into the intravascular space. This becomes important in the occasional patient who has intravascular volume depletion as assessed by your clinical examination, together with the interstitial fluid excess (i.e., edema).

In order to help shift fluid from the interstitium to the intravascular space, therefore, a logical choice is to administer IV albumin. Artificial plasma expanders (e.g., dextran, hetastarch) are high molecular weight glucose polymers that remain in the intravascular space because of their large size and serve the same purpose as albumin.

Remember that oncotic pull comes from albumin. It does not come from sodium, so NS is not an appropriate fluid to give in this situation; it does not come from red blood cells, so a blood transfusion is not an appropriate fluid to give.

Table 3-1. COMMONLY USED INTRAVENOUS FLUIDS

	Glucose (g/L)	Na (mmol/L)	Cl (mmol/L)	K (mmol/L)	Ca (mmol/L)	Lactate (mmol/L)	Approximate Osmolality (mOsm/L)
D5W	50	—	—	—	—	—	252
D10W	100	—	—	—	—	—	505
D20W	200	—	—	—	—	—	1010
D50W	500	—	—	—	—	—	2525
"⅔rds ⅓rd"	33	51	51	—	—	—	269
0.45% NaCl (½ NS)	—	77	77	—	—	—	154
0.9% NaCl (NS)	—	154	154	—	—	—	308
D5NS	50	154	154	—	—	—	560
Ringer's lactate	—	130	109	4	3	28	272

Albumin	—	145	145	Available in 5% concentrations (50, 250, or 500 ml) or 25% concentrations (20, 50, or 100 ml)
Fresh frozen plasma (FFP)				200 ml plasma that has been separated from whole blood and frozen within 6 hours of collection. FFP contains all coagulation factors.
Stored plasma				200 ml of plasma that has been separated from whole blood within 72 hours of collection. Contains all coagulation factors except V and VIII.

Note that albumin is available in two concentrations—5% and 25%. The 25% albumin is the preferred concentration when trying to effect a shift in fluid from the interstitial space to the intravascular space.

Unfortunately, albumin, plasma, and artificial plasma expanders are expensive, and their effect in removing edema fluid is transient. Hence, their continued use for this indication is controversial. Certainly, the best way to correct edema in a patient with a decreased intravascular volume but an excess of interstitital fluid is to correct the underlying cause of extravascular volume excess. In most cases, the cause is hypoproteinemia (e.g., malabsorption, liver disease, nephrotic syndrome, protein losing enteropathy).

In summary, most disorders of fluid balance can be treated logically and successfully by employing the simple principles of water and solute transfer across cell membranes. (See Table 3-1 for a listing of the commonly used IV fluids.)

PATIENT-RELATED PROBLEMS:
THE 20 COMMON CALLS

4

ABDOMINAL PAIN

Many patients complain of abdominal pain during their hospital stays. It is essential to distinguish the acute abdominal emergency from the recurrent non-emergency; the former requires urgent medical or surgical intervention, whereas the latter requires thorough, but less urgent, investigation.

PHONE CALL

Questions

1. **How severe is the pain?**
2. **Is the pain localized or generalized?**
3. **What are the vital signs?**
   Fever and abdominal pain are suggestive of intra-abdominal infection or inflammation.
4. **Is this a new problem?**
5. **Is the pain acute or chronic?**
6. **Is there any associated nausea, vomiting, or diarrhea?**
   Nausea and vomiting associated with acute abdominal pain suggest small bowel obstruction, gastric outlet obstruction, or biliary colic. Diarrhea and abdominal pain suggest inflammatory, ischemic, or infectious bowel disease.
7. **What was the reason for admission?**

Orders

If the abdominal pain is mild, ask the RN to phone immediately if the pain becomes worse before you are able to assess the patient.

Inform RN

"Will arrive at bedside in . . . minutes."

Abdominal pain of acute onset, severe abdominal pain, or pain associated with fever or hypotension requires you to see the patient immediately. Mild recurrent abdominal pain is a less urgent problem and may be attended to in an hour or two if other patient problems of higher priority exist.

ELEVATOR THOUGHTS (What causes abdominal pain?)

The causes of *localized abdominal pain* are numerous. A useful system for approaching the problem is "diagnosis by location." Figure 4–1 illustrates a differential diagnosis by location.

The causes of *generalized abdominal pain* are fewer. Disorders' producing either localized pain or generalized pain are indicated by an asterisk. Additional causes of generalized abdominal pain alone are listed in the key to Figure 4–1.

Key to Figure 4–1. Differential Diagnosis by Abdominal Quadrant

Right Upper Quadrant
    L—Liver (hepatitis, abscess, perihepatitis)
    GB—Gallbladder (cholelithiasis, choledocholithiasis)
    HF—Hepatic flexure (obstruction)
Left Lower Quadrant
    A—Appendix (appendicitis,* abscess)
Left Upper Quadrant
    Sp—Spleen (rupture, infarct, abscess)
    SF—Splenic flexure (obstruction)
Left Lower Quadrant
    LC—Left colon (diverticulitis, ischemic colitis)
Epigastrium
    H—Heart (myocardial infarction, pericarditis, aortic dissection)
    Lu—Lung (pneumonia, pleurisy)
    SA—Subphrenic abscess
    E—Esophagus (esophagitis)
    S—Stomach (peptic ulcer)
    P—Pancreas (pancreatitis)
    K—Kidney (pyelonephritis, renal colic (stones))
Hypogastrium
    K—Kidney (renal colic (stones))
    PA—Psoas abscess
    I—Intestine (infection,* obstruction,* inflammatory bowel disease*)
    O—Ovary (torsion of cyst, carcinoma)
    OT—Ovarian tube (ectopic pregnancy, salpingitis, endometriosis)
    B—Bladder (cystitis)
Generalized Abdominal Pain
    1. [See those marked with an asterisk.]
    2. Peritonitis (any cause)
    3. Diabetic ketoacidosis
    4. Sickle cell crisis
    5. Acute intermittent porphyria
    6. Acute adrenocortical insufficiency due to steroid withdrawal

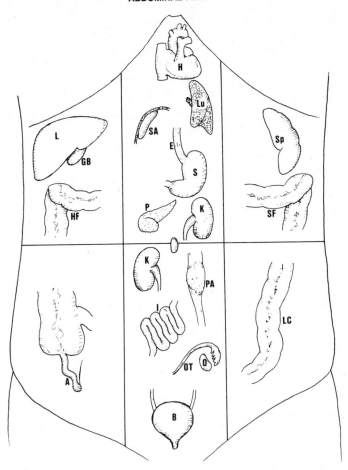

Figure 4–1. Differential diagnosis of abdominal pain by location. (See key on opposite page.)

MAJOR THREATS TO LIFE

- Perforated or ruptured viscus
- Ascending cholangitis
- Necrosis of viscus
- Exsanguinating hemorrhage

A perforated or ruptured viscus may result in hypovolemic shock (from third space losses), septic shock (from either chemical or bacterial peritonitis), or both. Progression of infection from the initial site (e.g., ascending cholangitis) to septic shock may occur rapidly, i.e., within hours of the patient's first presenting symptom.

Necrosis of a viscus, as in intussusception, volvulus, strangulated hernia, or ischemic colitis, can cause hypovolemic or septic shock and electrolyte and acid-base disturbances. Exsanguinating hemorrhage with hypovolemic shock may result from a ruptured ectopic pregnancy; from a splenic rupture; occasionally, from a liver or renal biopsy; or from a misdirected thoracentesis. Patients with myocardial infarction and aortic dissection occasionally present with abdominal pain. These diagnoses should be considered, especially if no local abdominal signs can be identified.

BEDSIDE

Quick Look Test

Does the patient look well (comfortable), sick (uncomfortable or distressed), or critical (about to die)?

Appearances are often deceptive in acute abdominal disease. If the patient has recently received narcotic analgesics or high dose steroids, he or she may appear well despite a serious underlying problem.

Patients suffering severe colic or intraperitoneal hemorrhage are often restless, in contrast to those suffering peritonitis who lie immobile, avoiding movement that exacerbates the pain. With peritonitis, patients may have their knees drawn up to reduce abdominal tension.

Airway and Vital Signs

What is the BP?

Hypotension associated with abdominal pain is an ominous sign suggestive of impending septic, hypovolemic, or hemorrhagic shock.

Are there orthostatic changes (lying and standing) in the BP and HR?

If there are postural changes, recheck the BP and HR with the patient standing. A drop in BP that is associated with an increased heart rate (> 15 beats/min) suggests volume depletion. A drop in BP without a change in the heart rate suggests autonomic dysfunction.

What is the temperature?

Fever associated with abdominal pain is suggestive of intra-abdominal infection or inflammation. However, the lack of a fever in the elderly patient or in the patient receiving an antipyretic or immunosuppressive drug does not rule out infection.

Selective History and Chart Review

Diagnosis is often dependent upon a careful history addressing (1) the pain at onset and its subsequent progression, (2) any associated symptoms, and (3) the past history.

Pain

Is the pain localized?

The maximum intensity of the pain can provide a clue to the site of origin (see Figure 4–1).

How is the pain characterized (e.g., severe or mild; burning or knife-like; constant or waxing and waning, as in colic)?

There are characteristic descriptions of pain associated with certain diseases as follows: the pain of peptic ulcer tends to be burning; that of a perforated ulcer is sudden, constant, and severe; that of biliary colic is sharp, constricting ("taking one's breath away"); that of acute pancreatitis is deep and agonizing; and that of obstructed bowel is "gripping," with intermittent worsening.

Did the pain develop gradually or suddenly?

The severe pain of "colic" (renal, biliary, or intestinal) develops in hours, whereas the pain of pancreatitis usually develops in days. An acute onset with fainting suggests perforation of a viscus, strangulation of the gut, ruptured ectopic pregnancy, torsion of an ovarian cyst, or biliary or renal colic.

Has the pain changed since its onset?

A ruptured viscus may initially be associated with localized pain, which subsequently shifts or becomes generalized with the development of chemical or bacterial peritonitis.

Does the pain radiate?

Radiation of the pain (i.e., referred pain) occurs to that dermatome or cutaneous area supplied by the same sensory cortical cells as the deep seated structure (Fig. 4–2). For example, the diaphragm is supplied by the cervical roots C3, C4, and C5. Many upper abdominal or lower thoracic conditions that cause irritation of the diaphragm refer pain to the cutaneous supply of C3, C4, and C5, i.e., the shoulder and the neck. The liver and gallbladder are derived from the right 7th and 8th thoracic segments; thus, biliary colic frequently refers pain to the inferior angle of the right scapula.

Are there any aggravating or relieving factors?

Pain that increases with meals, decreases with passage of bowel movements, or both suggests a hollow gut origin. An exception is pain from duodenal ulcer, which is often relieved by the ingestion

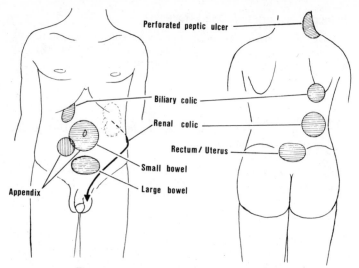

Figure 4–2. Common sites of referred pain.

of food. Pain that increases with inspiration suggests pleuritis or peritonitis; pain that is aggravated by micturition suggests a uro-genital cause.

Associated Symptoms

Is there any associated nausea or vomiting?

Vomiting occurring with the onset of pain frequently accompanies acute peritoneal irritation or perforation of a viscus. It is also commonly associated with acute pancreatitis or obstruction of any muscular hollow viscus. Pain relieved by vomiting suggests hollow gut origin (e.g., biliary colic) or pancreatic disease. Vomiting many hours after the onset of abdominal pain may be a clue to intestinal obstruction or ileus.

What is the nature of emesis?

Brown, feculent emesis is pathognomonic of bowel obstruction, either paralytic or mechanical. Frank blood is suggestive of an upper GI bleed. Vomiting food after fasting is consistent with gastric stasis or gastric outlet obstruction.

Is there any associated diarrhea?

Diarrhea and abdominal pain are seen in infectious gastroenteritis, ischemic colitis, appendicitis, and partial small bowel obstruction. Diarrhea alternating with constipation is a common symptom of diverticular disease.

Is there associated fever or chills?

Check the temperature record since admission. Check the medication sheet for antipyretic, steroid, or antibiotic drugs: fever may be masked by the administration of these medications.

Past History and Chart Review

Was the admitting diagnosis "abdominal pain NYD" in a previously healthy patient?

New, unremitting, undiagnosed severe abdominal pain suggests an abscess associated with a ruptured appendix or with a diverticular disease.

Is there a history of peptic ulcer disease or antacid ingestion?

Peptic ulcer disease is a chronic, recurring disease. History repeats itself!

Is there a history of blunt or penetrating trauma to the abdomen? Has there been a liver or kidney biopsy or a thoracentesis since admission?

A subcapsular hemorrhage of the spleen, liver, or kidney may result in hemorrhagic shock 1 to 3 days later.

Is there a history of alcohol abuse and ascites?

Spontaneous bacterial peritonitis must always be considered in the alcoholic patient with fever, abdominal pain, and ascites.

Is there a history of coronary or peripheral vascular disease?

Ischemic colitis is a consideration in the patient with atherosclerosis and abdominal pain.

If the patient is a premenopausal female, ask the date of the last normal menstrual period.

Abdominal pain associated with a missed period raises the possibility of an ectopic pregnancy. Hypotension in this situation suggests a ruptured ectopic pregnancy, a life-threatening situation.

Is there a history of previous abdominal surgery?

Adhesions are responsible for 70% of small bowel obstructions.

Is the patient anticoagulated?

Intra-abdominal hemorrhage may occur in the anticoagulated patient, especially if there is a history of peptic ulcer disease.

Is there a history of aspirin or NSAID, alcohol, or other ulcerogenic drug use?

Selective Physical Examination

VITALS	Repeat now
HEENT	Icterus (cholangitis, choledocholithiasis)
	Spider nevi (risk of spontaneous bacterial peritonitis if ascites is present)
RESP	Generalized or localized restriction of abdominal wall movement in respiration (localized or generalized peritoneal effusion)
	Stony dullness to percussion, decreased breath sounds, decreased tactile fremitus (pleural effusion)
	Dullness to percussion, diminished or bronchial breath sounds, crackles (consolidation and pneumonia)
CVS	Decreased JVP (volume depletion)
	Distant heart sounds (pericarditis)
	New onset of dysrhythmia, mitral insufficiency murmur, or S_4 (myocardial infarction)
ABD	Before examining the abdomen make sure your hands are warm and make sure the head of the bed is flat. It may be helpful to flex the patient's hips, in order to relax the abdominal wall. When examining for tenderness, begin in a non-painful region.
	Visible peristalsis (bowel obstruction)
	Bulging flanks (ascites)
	Caput medusa (Fig. 4–3) (portal hypertension and increased risk of spontaneous bacterial peritonitis)
	Loss of liver dullness (perforated viscus)
	Localized tenderness, masses (see Fig. 4–1)
	Rigid abdomen, guarding, rebound tenderness (peritonitis)
	Shifting dullness, fluid wave (ascites)
	Absent bowel sounds (paralytic ileus or bowel obstruction)
	Check all hernia orifices (strangulated hernia) (Fig. 4–4)
	Murphy's sign (cholecystitis) (Fig. 4–5)
	Psoas sign (retrocecal appendicitis, psoas abscess) (Fig. 4–6)
	Obturator sign (retrocecal appendicitis) (Fig. 4–7)
RECTAL	Tenderness (retrocecal appendicitis)
	Mass (rectal carcinoma)
	Rectal fissure (Crohn's disease)
	Stool positive for occult blood (ischemic colitis, peptic ulcer)
PELVIC	Tenderness (ectopic pregnancy, ovarian cyst, or pelvic inflammatory disease)
	Mass (ovarian cyst or tumor)

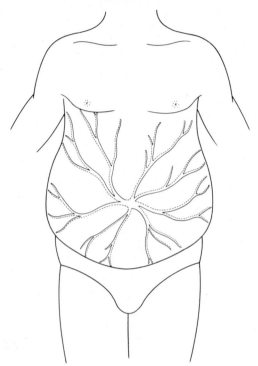

Figure 4–3. Caput medusae.

Management

Hypovolemic Shock

Hypovolemic shock from any cause requires immediate volume replacement and surgical consultation.

Rapid volume repletion using normal saline or Ringer's lactate (500 ml IV as rapidly as possible, followed by an IV rate titrated to the JVP and vital signs).

Blood should be drawn for a stat crossmatch for 4 to 6 units of packed RBCs, Hb, PT, PTT, and platelet count. If hemorrhage-induced shock is suspected, packed RBCs should be given in place of or in addition to the crystalloid NS or Ringer's lactate, as soon as the crossmatch has been completed.

Baseline values of the following should be determined: electrolytes, urea, creatinine, random blood glucose, amylase, CBC, and manual differential.

Urgent surgical consultation is required. Ensure the patient is NPO. Consider inserting an NG tube if the patient is vomiting.

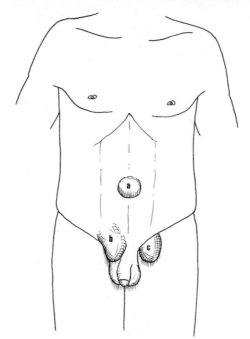

Figure 4–4. Hernial orifices. a = Umbilical hernia, b = inguinal hernia, and c = femoral hernia.

Septic Shock

Septic shock from any cause also requires immediate volume replacement, appropriate cultures, and empiric, broad-spectrum antibiotics. Early surgical consultation is required for drainage where indicated.

Initiate volume repletion using normal saline or Ringer's lactate, 500 ml IV as rapidly as possible, followed by an IV rate titrated to the JVP and the vital signs. Order three radiographic views of the abdomen as follows: (A/P abdomen supine and erect or lateral decubitus and P/A chest erect).

Toxic megacolon is manifested by an increase in the diameter of the mid-transverse colon (> 7 cm) and a mucosal pattern of thumbprinting or thickening. This condition is a medical or surgical emergency. Look for air under the diaphragm in the chest film or between the viscera and subcutaneous tissue in the lateral decubitus film; this sign is indicative of a perforated viscus.

Draw blood for a stat CBC, manual differential, and blood cultures ×2. In addition, baseline values of the following should be determined: electrolytes, urea, creatinine, blood glucose, amylase, PT, and aPTT.

Specimens for Gram's stain, culture, and sensitivity testing

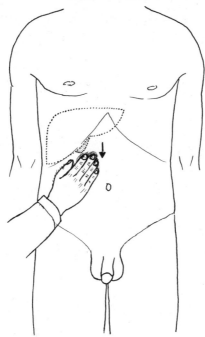

Figure 4–5. Murphy's sign. A positive Murphy's sign is manifested by pain and "inspiratory arrest" when the patient takes a deep breath while the examiner applies pressure against the abdominal wall in the region of the gallbladder.

should be obtained immediately from sputum, if available; urine, which may require in/out catheterization; and wounds. If there is ascites, an immediate diagnostic paracentesis should be performed.

Once culture have been obtained, empiric, broad-spectrum antibiotics (ampicillin, an aminoglycoside, plus metronidazole or cefoxitin) should be started immediately, to treat infection due to

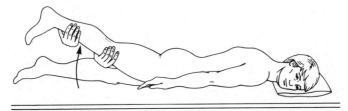

Figure 4–6. Psoas sign. A positive psoas sign is manifested by abdominal pain in response to passive hip flexion. (The test may also be performed with the patient lying on his or her side.)

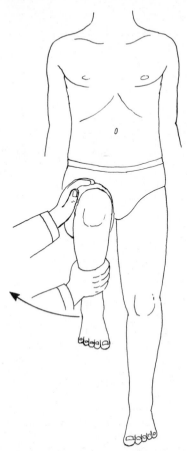

Figure 4–7. A positive obturator sign is manifested by abdominal pain in response to passive internal rotation of the right hip from the 90-degree hip/knee flexion position.

coliforms and gut anaerobes.

Urgent surgical consultation is required. However, medical re-suscitation with fluids and antibiotics must be started prior to surgical drainage. Ensure the patient is NPO.

If hypovolemia and septic shock are not present, most causes of abdominal pain will require the following baseline investigations unless recent results are available:

- Three radiographic views of the abdomen (A/P abdomen supine and erect or decubitus and P/A chest)

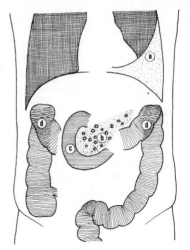

Figure 4–8. Radiographic features of pancreatitis. a = Left pleural effusion, b = calcification within the pancreas, c = sentinel loop, and d = colonic distention.

■ Electrolytes, urea, creatinine, blood glucose, amylase, CBC, and manual differential.

Pancreatitis

Pancreatitis should be suspected in the alcoholic patient with abdominal pain but with no evidence of an upper GI bleed or ascites. The abdominal x-ray films may reveal a sentinel loop, A colonic distention, a left pleural effusion, or a calcification within the pancreas (Fig. 4–8). An elevated amylase level supports the diagnosis, but a normal amylase level does not exclude the possibility of pancreatitis. The patient should be NPO. IV fluids with NS should be ordered to replace any losses. Narcotic analgesia usually will be required. *Meperidine* (Demerol) 50 to 150 mg IM or SC q3 to 4hr PRN is the drug of choice, since morphine can cause spasm of Oddi's sphincter. If the patient develops a fever, an abdominal ultrasound scan should be ordered to search for a possible pancreatic pseudocyst.

Intra-abdominal Abscesses

Intra-abdominal abscesses will require delineation by either ultrasound or CT scan; this can be arranged in the morning provided the patient is otherwise stable. Subphrenic and psoas abscesses will require decompression. Hepatic abscesses may be drained percutaneously under ultrasound guidance or surgically. Splenic abscesses usually require splenectomy.

Peptic Ulcer Disease or Gastritis

Cases of suspected peptic ulcer disease or gastritis should be considered for endoscopy. H2 blockers should be started as follows:

cimetidine (Tagamet) 300 mg IV or PO q6 to 8hr (300 mg IV BID in renal failure) or *ranitidine* (Zantac) 50 mg IV q8hr or 150 mg PO BID (50 mg PO or IV BID in renal failure). Antacids are contraindicated if endoscopy is to be performed, since antacids coat the lining of the stomach, obscuring the endoscopist's view of mucosal lesions.

Pyelonephritis

Pyelonephritis requires empiric IV antibiotics (ampicillin and an aminoglycoside), until the specific organism has been identified.

Renal Stones

Patients with renal stones may be managed medically with narcotic analgesics after the diagnosis has been confirmed with an IVP. Surgical removal or lithotripsy may be required if the stone has not passed within a few days, if the IVP reveals a staghorn calculus, or if an associated persistent infection is present.

Infectious Gastroenteritis

Infectious gastroenteritis may require specific antibiotics if the stool culture results reveal a bacterial cause. Viral gastroenteritis is treated supportively with IV fluids. *Clostridium difficile* infection should be suspected in any patient developing diarrhea during or after a course of antibiotics. Sigmoidoscopy may reveal a characteristic pseudomembrane, in which case *metronidazole* 500 mg PO q6hr or *vancomycin* 125 to 500 mg PO q6hr may be instituted prior to confirmation by *C. difficile* culture or toxin assay.

Ovarian Cyst, Tumor, or Salpingitis

These are best managed by referral to a gynecologist.

5

CHEST PAIN

In developed countries, where coronary artery disease is the leading cause of death, it is not surprising that when a patient presents complaining of "chest pain," you will wonder whether the patient is having angina or, worse yet, a heart attack. There are, however, several other equally serious causes of chest pain that may go undiagnosed if not specifically looked for. In the assessment of chest pain, history-taking is your most powerful tool.

PHONE CALL

Questions

1. **How severe is the pain?**
2. **What are the vital signs?**
3. **What was the reason for admission?**
4. **Does the patient have a past history of myocardial infarction or angina? If yes, is the pain similar to their usual angina or previous infarction?**

Orders

1. ECG stat if myocardial ischemia is suspected.
2. Oxygen by face mask or nasal prongs at 10 L/min. If the patient is a CO_2 retainer, you will have to be cautious when giving oxygen (maximum FIO_2 0.28 by mask or 2 L/min by nasal prongs).
3. Nitroglycerin 0.3 mg SL q5min provided the systolic BP is > 90 mm Hg.
4. IV D5W TKVO unless already in place.
5. ABG set to be available at the bedside.
6. Ask the RN to take the patient's chart to the bedside.

Inform RN

"Will arrive at bedside in . . . minutes."

Most causes of chest pain are diagnosed by history. It is impossible to obtain an accurate and relevant history by speaking to the RN over the phone; the history must be taken first hand from the patient. Because some causes of chest pain represent medical emergencies, the patient should be assessed immediately.

ELEVATOR THOUGHTS (What causes chest pain?)

CARDIAC	Angina
	Myocardial infarction
	Aortic dissection
	Pericarditis
RESP	Pulmonary embolus or infarction
	Pneumothorax
	Pleuritis (+/− pneumonia)
GI	Esophageal spasm, reflux, candidiasis
	Peptic ulcer disease
MSS	Costochondritis
	Rib fracture

MAJOR THREAT TO LIFE

- Myocardial ischemia
- Aortic dissection
- Pneumothorax
- Pulmonary embolus

Cardiogenic shock or fatal dysrhythmias may occur as a result of myocardial infarction. Aortic dissection may result in death from cardiac tamponade or myocardial infarction. Pneumothorax and pulmonary embolism cause hypoxia.

BEDSIDE

Quick Look Test

Does the patient look well (comfortable), sick (uncomfortable or distressed), or critical (about to die)?

Most patients with chest pain from myocardial infarction or severe ischemia look sick. If the patient looks well, suspect esophagitis or a musculoskeletal problem, such as costochondritis.

Airway and Vital Signs

What is the BP?

Most patients with chest pain will have normal BP. Hypotension may be seen with myocardial infarction, massive pulmonary embolism, or tension pneumothorax. Hypertension, occurring in association with myocardial ischemia or aortic dissection, should be treated urgently (see Chapter 13, page 119).

What is the HR?

Does the patient have tachycardia? Severe chest pain of any cause may result in sinus tachycardia. Heart rates > 100 min should alert you to the possibility of tachydysrhythmia, such as atrial fibrillation, SVT, or ventricular tachycardia, which may require immediate cardioversion.

Does the patient have bradycardia? Bradycardia in a patient with chest pain may represent sinus or AV nodal ischemia (as may be seen with myocardial infarction) or beta blockade due to drugs. Immediate treatment of bradycardia is not required unless the patient is hypotensive (see Chapter 15, page 131).

Management I

Is the patient receiving oxygen?

Ensure that the patient is receiving oxygen at an appropriate concentration.

Does the patient have chest pain now?

Chest pain and systolic BP > 90 mm Hg

- If the last dose of sublingual nitroglycerin was given > 5 minutes ago, order another dose immediately.
- If the patient was receiving 0.3 mg and it made no difference in the relief chest pain, increase the dose to 0.6 mg.
- If the pain continues despite three doses of nitroglycerin, order 10 mg (1 ml) of morphine to be drawn into a syringe diluted with 9 ml of NS. Give the *morphine* in 2 to 4 mg aliquots IV until the pain is relieved, provided the systolic BP is > 90 mm Hg. Morphine sulfate may cause hypotension or respiratory depression. Take the BP and RR before each dose is given. If necessary, *naloxone hydrochloride* (Narcan) 0.2 to 2 mg IV or SC may be given q5min to a total of 10 mg to reverse these side effects. Nausea or vomiting may also occur and can usually be controlled with *dimenhydrinate* (Dramamine, Gravol) 25 mg IV or 50 mg PO q4hr PRN.
- If the chest pain requires the administration of morphine arrange for transfer to the ICU/CCU as soon as possible

Chest pain and systolic BP < 90 mm Hg

- What is the patient's normal BP? If the systolic BP is normally 90 mm Hg, you may proceed cautiously with sublingual nitroglycerin 0.3 mg, as described, provided there is no further drop in the BP.
- If the hypotension is an acute change, establish IV access immediately with a large bore IV (size 16 if possible). Refer to Chapter 15, page 133, for management of hypotension.

If the patient looks sick or critical
Draw ABG sample.
Establish IV access using D5W if not already done.

Read the ECG
Coronary artery disease is common. Many patients seen at night with chest pain will have myocardial ischemia. Remember, a normal ECG does not rule out the possibility of angina or myocardial infarction.

Selective History and Chart Review

How does the patient describe the pain? Is the pain the same as the patient's usual angina?
Crushing, squeezing, vise-like pain or pressure is characteristic of myocardial infarction. Severe tearing or ripping pain is characteristic of an aortic dissection.

Does the pain radiate?
Radiation of pain to the back suggests myocardial ischemia or aortic dissection distal to the left subclavian artery. Dissection proximal to the left subclavian artery causes non-radiating anterior chest pain. Review the chest x-ray as soon as possible, looking specifically for a widened mediastinum. Suspected aortic dissection requires you to proceed urgently with the appropriate investigation and management (see page 119).

Is there any associated nausea, vomiting, diaphoresis, or lightheadedness?
Cardiogenic nausea and vomiting are associated with larger myocardial infarctions but do not suggest a particular location as previously thought.

Is the chest pain worse with deep breathing or coughing?
Pleuritic chest pain suggests pleuritis, pneumothorax, rib fracture, pericarditis, pulmonary embolism, pneumonia, or costochondritis.

Selective Physical Examination

VITALS	Repeat now.
HEENT	Blindness (aortic dissection)
	White exudate in oral cavity or pharynx (thrush with possible concomitant esophageal candidiasis)
RESP	Crackles (CHF secondary to acute MI or pulmonary embolism)
	Consolidation and pleural effusion (pulmonary infarction or pneumonia)

CVS	Unequal upper limb BP or diminished femoral pulses (aortic dissection)
	Elevated JVP (right ventricular failure secondary to MI or cor pulmonale)
	Right ventricular heave (cor pulmonale)
	Left ventricular heave (CHF)
	Loud P_2 (cor pulmonale), S_3 (CHF)
	Mitral insufficiency murmur (papillary muscle dysfunction)
	Aortic insufficiency murmur (dissection at base of aortic root)
	Pericardial rub (pericarditis)
	Pericardial rubs are biphasic or triphasic scratching sounds that vary with position.
ABD	Guarding, rebound tenderness (perforated ulcer)
	Epigastric tenderness (peptic ulcer disease)
	Generalized abdominal pain (mesenteric infarction from aortic dissection)
CNS	Hemiplegia (aortic dissection)

Management II

Angina. If *angina* has been relieved with 1 to 3 nitroglycerin tablets, review the precipitating cause. An adjustment in the anti-anginal medication may be required and should be made in consultation with your resident and attending physician. However, if the angina occurred at rest, or this is the first episode of angina, the patient should be assessed by the ICU/CCU staff regardless of whether the pain was relieved with ≤ 3 nitroglycerin tablets.

If the angina required more than 3 doses of nitroglycerin, serial cardiac enzyme tests and ECGs should be ordered. If the clinical impression is of possible myocardial infarction, the patient should be transferred to the ICU/CCU for continuous ECG monitoring.

If the angina required IV morphine, the patient should be transferred to the ICU/CCU and treated as having a possible myocardial infarction.

Myocardial Infarction. If a *myocardial infarction* is suspected by history or electrocardiographic changes (see page 289), the patient should be transferred to the ICU/CCU as soon as possible. In addition to morphine, myocardial ischemia may require treatment with IV nitroglycerin or beta blockers. The patient should also be evaluated for possible thrombolytic therapy.

Aortic Dissection. Suspicion of *aortic dissection* requires urgent investigation and management as follows:

1. Arrange for an urgent CT scan of the thorax.
2. Draw blood for a stat crossmatch for 6 to 8 units of packed

RBCs on hold, electrolytes, urea, creatinine, glucose, CBC and differential, PT, and aPTT.
3. Review the ECG for evidence of an acute MI; this finding suggests aortic dissection involving the coronary ostia.
4. The patient should be transferred to the ICU/CCU as soon as possible for careful control of blood pressure (see Chapter 13, page 119).
5. Surgical consultation should be obtained early when the diagnosis of dissection had been entertained. The diagnosis can be confirmed with aortography.

Pericarditis. Patients with suspected *pericarditis* should have nonurgent echocardiograms to look for pericardial effusions or signs of hemodynamic compromise. *Indomethacin* (Indocin) 50 mg PO TID or *aspirin* 650 mg PO QID are helpful.

NSAIDs are contraindicated in the patient who has the syndrome of aspirin sensitivity, nasal polyps, and bronchospasm, in the patient who is anticoagulated, or in the patient who has active peptic ulcer disease. Because of their sodium retaining properties, caution should be used in giving NSAIDs to patients in CHF. NSAIDs should also be used with caution in patients with renal insufficiency, as these drugs may inhibit renal prostaglandins which are responsible for maintaining renal perfusion in those with prerenal conditions. Sulindac (Clinoril) may not have this effect.

Pulmonary Embolus. The management of *pulmonary embolus* is discussed in Chapter 20, page 210.

Pneumothorax. A *pneumothorax* may require chest tube drainage depending upon its size. If the patient develops a tension pneumothorax, immediate treatment is necessary to relieve the pressure using a size 16 gauge intravenous catheter as described on page 146.

Pneumonia. Suggested antibiotics for *pneumonia* are discussed in Chapter 20, page 212, and should be chosen according to the Gram's stain results and patient's characteristics.

Esophagitis. *Esophagitis* may be treated with antacids. Choose carefully. Magnesium containing antacids (Gelusil, Maalox) may cause diarrhea, whereas antacids containing solely aluminum (Amphojel, Basaljel) may cause constipation. Don't substitute one GI complaint for another! *Gelusil* 30 to 60 ml 1 hr and 3 hr PC meals and qhs is a standard antacid order. More frequent doses may be required if the pain is severe. Elevation of the head of the bed may also be helpful.

Esophageal candidiasis will not respond to antacids! Immunocompromised patients may experience severe chest pain from this problem. Diagnosis should be confirmed by endoscopy. Treatment with *nystatin* (Mycostatin) 400,000 to 600,000 units PO (swish and swallow) QID is usually effective. However, in immunocompromised patients (e.g., those with AIDS) *clotrimazole* (Canesten) 10 mg troche PO QID or *ketaconazole* 200 to 400 mg PO daily are more effective.

Peptic Ulcer. A patient with *suspected peptic ulcer disease* should be referred to a gastroenterologist for a possible endoscopic evaluation in the morning.

Costochondritis. *Costochondritis* may be treated with an NSAID, such as *naproxen* (Naprosyn), 250 mg PO BID. NSAIDs are contraindicated in the patient who has the syndrome of aspirin sensitivity, nasal polyps, and bronchospasm, in the patient who is anticoagulated, or in the patient who has active peptic ulcer disease. Because of their sodium retaining properties, caution should be used in giving NSAIDs to patients in CHF. NSAIDs should also be used with caution in patients with renal insufficiency, as these drugs can inhibit renal prostaglandins which are responsible for maintaining renal perfusion in patients with prerenal conditions. Sulindac (Clinoril) may not have this effect.

6

CONFUSION

Confusion is a common problem in hospitalized patients. Unfortunately, the terms delirium, toxic psychosis, acute brain syndrome, and acute confusional state are often used interchangeably to refer to any cause of confusion. When the term metabolic encephalopathy is used, it implies that the confusion is not due to psychiatric disorders or structural intracranial lesions.

The two recommended terms are delirium and dementia. *Delirium* is characterized by restlessness; agitation; clouding of consciousness; and, in some patients, bizarre behavior, hallucinations, delusions, and illusions. *Dementia* refers to a state of irreversible loss of memory and a global cognitive deficit. The level of consciousness is an important distinguishing feature between delirium and dementia; delirium is characterized by a clouding of consciousness (a decreased clarity of awareness of the environment), whereas dementia is associated with a normal level of consciousness.

PHONE CALL

Questions

1. Clarify the situation. **In what way is the patient confused?**
2. **What are the vital signs?**
3. **Has there been a change in the level of consciousness?**
4. **Have there been previous episodes of confusion?**
5. **What was the reason for admission?**
6. **Is the patient diabetic?**
7. **How old is the patient?**
   A 30-year-old patient is much more likely to have a serious yet reversible cause of confusion than an 80-year-old patient receiving multiple medications.
8. **What medication is the patient receiving?**

Orders

1. Blood glucose, Chemstrip, or Glucometer reading. Hypoglycemia is a rapidly reversible cause of confusion.

Inform RN

"Will arrive at the bedside in . . . minutes."
Confusion in association with fever, decrease in the level of

consciousness, or acute agitation (i.e., patient "out-of-control") requires you to see the patient immediately.

ELEVATOR THOUGHTS (What causes confusion?)

CNS (Intracranial)

1. Dementia
   Alzheimer's disease (80 to 90% of all dementias)
   Multi-infarct dementia
   Parkinson's disease
   Normal pressure hydrocephalus
2. Malignancy (primary CNS tumor, CNS metastasis, paraneoplastic syndrome)
3. Head trauma (subdural and epidural hematoma, concussion)
4. Post-ictal state
5. Stroke
6. Hypertensive encephalopathy
7. Wernicke's encephalopathy (thiamine deficiency)
8. B_{12} deficiency

Systemic

Drugs

1. Alcohol withdrawal. Confusion in the alcoholic patient may occur when the patient is intoxicated, during early withdrawal, or later as part of delirium tremens.
2. Narcotic and sedative drug excess or withdrawal. Even "normal" doses of these drugs frequently cause confusion in the elderly.
3. NSAIDs including aspirin
4. Anti-hypertensives (methyldopa, beta blockers)
5. Psychotropic medications (tricyclic antidepressants, lithium, phenothiazines, MAO inhibitors, benzodiazepines)
6. Miscellaneous (steroids, cimetidine, antihistamines, anticholinergics)

Organ Failure

1. Respiratory failure (hypoxia, CO_2 retention, fat embolism syndrome)
2. Renal failure
3. Liver failure (hepatic encephalopathy)
4. CHF, hypertensive encephalopathy

Metabolic

1. Hyperglycemia, hypoglycemia
2. Hypernatremia, hyponatremia
3. Hypercalcemia

Endocrine
1. Hyperthyroidism or hypothyroidism
2. Hyperadrenocorticism or hypoadrenocorticism

Infection or Inflammation
1. Meningitis, encephalitis, brain abscess
2. Lyme disease
3. Cerebral vasculitis (SLE, polyarteritis nodosa)

Psychiatric Disorders
1. Mania, depression
2. Schizophrenia

MAJOR THREAT TO LIFE

- Subdural or epidural hematoma
- Delirium tremens
- Meningitis
- Septic shock

Patients with a subdural or epidural hematoma may present initially with confusion. Untreated delirium tremens patients can suffer a mortality rate of up to 15%. Meningitis needs to be recognized early if antibiotic medication is to be effective. Unrecognized infection from any source can result in septic shock, especially in the elderly patient who may not manifest the typical features of an infection.

BEDSIDE

Quick Look Test

Does the patient look well (comfortable), sick (uncomfortable or distressed), or critical (about to die)?
Most patients with delirium look sick, whereas most patients with dementia look well.

Airway, Vital Signs, and Chemstrip Results

Is the patient receiving oxygen?
An FIO_2 of > 0.28 given to a patient with COPD may depress the respiratory center, resulting in confusion from hypercarbia.

What is the BP?
Hypertensive encephalopathy is rare; diastolic BP is usually

> 120 mm Hg. Confusion in association with a systolic BP < 90 mm Hg may be due to impaired cerebral perfusion secondary to shock. Drug overdose, adrenal insufficiency, and hyponatremia are metabolic causes that should be considered in the hypotensive, confused patient.

What is the HR?

A tachycardia suggests sepsis, delirium tremens, hyperthyroidism, or hypoglycemia, but it may also be seen in any agitated, anxious patient.

What is the temperature?

Fever suggests infection, delirium tremens, cerebral vasculitis, or fat embolism syndrome.

What is the respiratory rate?

Confusion in association with tachypnea should alert you to the possibility of hypoxia. Tachypnea with confusion and petechiae in a young patient with a femoral fracture is a classic presentation of fat embolism syndrome.

What is the blood glucose result?

Hypoglycemia is most commonly seen in the patient with diabetes mellitus who has received the usual insulin dose but has not eaten. Rarely, a wrong dose of insulin, a surreptitious insulin use, or an insulinoma is the cause (See Chapter 26, page 262, for the management of hypoglycemia and page 259, for the management of hyperglycemia.)

Selective Physical Examination I

HEENT   Nuchal rigidity (meningitis)
         Papilledema (hypertensive encephalopathy, intracranial mass)
         Pupil size and symmetry
             Dilated pupils suggest increased sympathetic outflow, such as may be seen in delirium tremens, whereas pinpoint pupils suggest narcotic excess or recent application of constricting eye drops.
         Palpate the skull for fractures, hematomas, and lacerations (subdural or epidural hematoma, concussion).
         Hemotympanum or blood in the ear canal (basal skull fracture).

NEURO   A detailed mental status examination is required in the assessment of the confused patient. However, if the patient has a decreased level of consciousness, is agitated or uncooperative, not all the categories discussed subsequently will be appropriate.

Mental status

General appearance—behavior and attitude.

Level of consciousness—alert, drowsy

Orientation—time, place, and person

Attention—digit recall

Speech—language deficit

Mood, affect—depressed, agitated, restless

Form of thought—flight of ideas, circumstantiality, loosening of associations, perseveration

Thought content—delusions, concrete thinking

Perceptions—illusions, hallucinations (auditory, visual)

Memory—immediate = digit repetition, recall of four objects after 5 minutes; recent = questions about the past 24 hours; remote = birthday, name of home town

Intellectual function—name the past three heads of state of the country

Calculation—serial 7's or serial 3's

Judgment—test hypothetical situations

A full neurologic examination is required (within the limits posed by the mental status examination). Is there any tremor (delirium tremens, Parkinson's disease)?

Is there any *asymmetry* of pupils, visual fields, eye movement, limbs, tone, reflexes, or plantars?

Asymmetry suggests structural brain disease.

Management I

Bacterial Meningitis. If there is suspicion of *bacterial meningitis,* refer immediately to Chapter 9, page 69, for further investigation and management.

Intracranial Lesion. *A structural intracranial lesion* (e.g., stroke, tumor, subdural hematoma, or epidural hematoma) should be suspected in the patient with new findings of asymmetry on neurologic examination. An urgent CT head scan will help define the intracranial lesion. Prompt referral to a neurosurgeon will be required for a subdural or epidural hematoma and for a cerebellar hemorrhage.

Delirium Tremens. *Delirium tremens* (confusion, fever, tachycar-

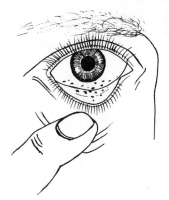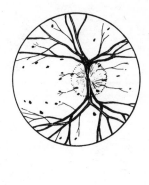

Figure 6–1. Conjunctival and fundal petechiae seen in fat embolism syndrome.

dia, dilated pupils, diaphoresis) and alcohol withdrawal need to be treated urgently with sedation. Benzodiazepines are of proven benefit. The loading dose of *diazepam* (Valium) is 5 to 10 mg IV at a rate of 2 to 5 mg/min q30 to 60 min, until the patient is sedated (i.e., drowsy but rouses when stimulated). The maintenance dose is 10 to 20 mg PO QID, with subsequent tapering. Alternatively, *Chlordiazepoxide* 100 mg PO QID for several days, with subsequent gradual tapering of the dose, can be used.

Thiamine. *Thiamine* 100 mg PO, IM, or IV daily for up to 3 days should be given to prevent the development of Wernicke's encephalopathy. IV D5NS should be given to correct volume depletion, once the initial dose of thiamine has been given.

Selective Physical Examination II

(Are there other correctable causes of confusion?)

VITALS	Repeat now.
HEENT	Conjunctival and fundal petechiae (fat embolism syndrome) (see Fig. 6–1)
	Lacerated tongue or cheek (post-ictal)
	Goiter (hyperthyroidism or hypothyroidism)
RESP	Cyanosis (hypoxia)
	Barrel chest (COPD with hypoxia or hypercarbia)
	Bibasilar crackles (CHF with hypoxia)
CVS	Elevated JVP ⎫
	S$_3$ ⎬ (CHF)
	Pitting edema ⎭

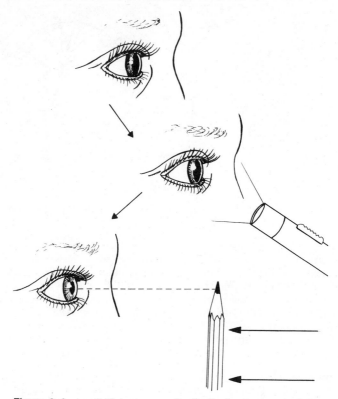

Figure 6–2. Argyll Robertson pupils. Pupils do not react to light, but they accommodate.

ABD   Costovertebral angle tenderness (pyelonephritis)
        Liver, spleen, or kidney tenderness (infection)
        Guarding, rebound tenderness (intra-abdominal infection)
        Shifting dullness, dilated superficial veins, caput medusa (liver failure)
NEURO   Argyll Robertson pupils, i.e., accommodate but do not react to light (syphilis) (Fig. 6–2)
        Cranial nerve palsies (Lyme disease)
        Asterixis, constructional apraxia (liver failure) (Fig. 6–3)
SKIN   Axillary fold, neck, upper chest petechiae (fat embolism syndrome)

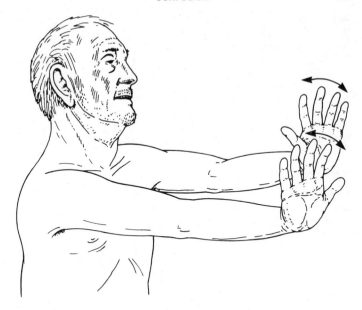

Tests of Constructional Apraxia
a. Copy the following:

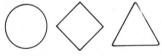

b. Draw a house or a clock face
c. Write signature

Figure 6–3. *Top,* Asterixis. Wrist "flapping" seen when the arms are outstretched. *Bottom,* Tests of constructional apraxia.

Selective History and Chart Review

What drugs is the patient receiving?

Remember, even the "usual" doses of some drugs can cause confusion in the elderly.

Is there a history of alcohol abuse?

It is important to establish when alcohol was last taken, since withdrawal symptoms are unlikely after 1 week of abstinence.

Examine the most recent laboratory test results for those that may indicate the reason for confusion in the patient. Not all of the tests listed subsequently will be available or pertinent.

- Blood glucose (hypoglycemia, hyperglycemia)
- Urea, creatinine (renal failure)

- Liver function (liver failure)
- Sodium (hyponatremia, hypernatremia)
- Calcium (hypercalcemia)
- Hb, MCV, RBC morphology (anemia with oval macrocytes suggests B_{12} or folate deficiency)
- WBC and differential (infection)
- ABG (hypoxia or CO_2 retention)
- T_4, TSH (hyperthyroidism, hypothyroidism)
- ANA, rheumatoid factor, ESR, C3, C4 (vasculitis)
- Drug levels (digoxin, lithium, aspirin, anti-epileptic drugs)

Management II

Drugs. If the confusion is *secondary to drugs,* stop the medication. If reversal of postoperative narcotic depression is indicated give *naloxone* (Narcan) 0.2 to 2.0 mg IV, IM, or SC q5 min (maximum total dose 10 mg) until the desired improved level of consciousness is achieved. Maintenance doses q1 to 2hr may be required to maintain reversal of the CNS depression. Naloxone should be used with caution in patients known to be physically dependent on opiates.

Dementia. *Dementia* is a diagnosis of exclusion. The following investigations are required to rule out a treatable cause of dementia:

- CBC, electrolytes, urea, creatinine
- Calcium, phosphorus
- Liver function tests
- Serum B_{12}, T_4
- STS
- CT head scan

Renal and Hepatic Failure. In end-stage *renal* and *liver failure* ensure the problem has not been compounded by hepatotoxic or nephrotoxic medications. Aggressive treatment of the renal failure (dialysis) or the liver failure (lactulose, neomycin) should be undertaken where indicated.

Hyponatremia or Hypernatremia. For the management of *hyponatremia* or *hypernatremia,* refer to Chapter 28.

Hypercalcemia. For the management of *hypercalcemia,* see Chapter 24.

B_{12} Deficiency. *B_{12} deficiency* needs to be confirmed by RBC morphology. If oval macrocytes are seen, order a RBC folate level and a serum B_{12} level.

Mania, Depression, or Schizophrenia. *Suspected mania, depression,* or *schizophrenia* requires psychiatric consultation for confirmation of diagnosis. Agitation in a confused patient may require *haloperidol* (Haldol) 1 to 5 mg PO or IM q4 to 6h.

Cerebral Vasculitis. *Cerebral vasculitis* is rare. High dose steroid therapy is the currently accepted treatment.

Fat Embolism. *Fat embolism syndrome* can have a mortality rate of up to 8%. The mainstay of treatment is oxygen therapy. If the patient requires an FIO_2 of > 0.5, then transfer to the ICU/CCU for probable intubation and mechanical ventilation with PEEP (positive end-expiratory pressure) is recommended.

7

DECREASED URINE OUTPUT

Decreased urine output is a frequently seen problem on both medical and surgical services. Proper management of these patients calls upon your skills in assessing volume status.

PHONE CALL

Questions

1. **How much urine has been passed in the last 24 hours?**
   Urine output less than 400 ml/day (< 20 ml/hr) = oliguria.
2. **What are the vital signs?**
3. **What was the reason for admission?**
4. **Is the patient complaining of abdominal pain?**
   Abdominal pain is a clue to the possible presence of a distended bladder as may be seen with bladder outlet obstruction.
5. **Is the patient anuric?**
   Anuria suggests a mechanical obstruction of the bladder outlet or a blocked Foley's catheter.
6. **Does the patient have a Foley's catheter?**
   If the patient has a Foley's catheter in place, the urine output assessment usually can be assumed to be accurate. If not, you will have to ensure that the total volume of voided urine has been collected and measured.

Orders

1. If a Foley's catheter is in place and the patient is anuric, ask the nurse to flush the catheter with 20 to 30 ml NS to ensure patency. A Foley's catheter clogged with sediment is a common problem and a satisfying one to treat before beginning a more detailed investigation for decreased urine output.
2. Serum electrolytes, urea, creatinine. A serum potassium level of > 5.5 mmol/L indicates that hyperkalemia is present. This is the most serious complication of renal insufficiency. A serum HCO_3 measurement < 20 mmol/L suggests metabolic acidosis due to renal insufficiency. A serum $HCO_3 < 15$ mmol/L should prompt you to determine the arterial pH. Elevations in serum urea and creatinine levels can be used as guidelines to assess the degree of renal insufficiency present.

Inform RN

"Will arrive at bedside in . . . minutes."

Provided the patient is not in pain and a recent serum potassium level is not elevated, assessment of decreased urine output can wait 1 or 2 hours, if other problems of higher priority exist.

ELEVATOR THOUGHTS (What causes decreased urine output?)

Prerenal Causes	Volume depletion
	CHF
	NSAIDs
	Hepatorenal syndrome
Renal Causes	Glomerular problems
	Nephritic syndromes (SLE, Wegener's, Goodpasture's, vasculitis)
	Nephritis syndromes (SLE, amyloidosis, IDDM)
	Tubulo-interstitial problems
	Acute tubular necrosis due to hypotension
	Acute interstitial nephritis due to penicillin, NSAIDs, or diuretics
	Chronic interstitial disease (hypertension, IDDM)
	Nephrotoxins
	Exogenous (aminoglycosides, IV contrast materials, cancer chemotherapy)
	Endogenous (myoglobin, uric acid, oxalate, amyloid, Bence Jones protein)
	Vascular Problems
	Atheromatous embolus
	Renal artery thrombosis
Post-renal Causes (obstruction)	Bilateral ureteric obstruction (e.g., stones, clots, sloughed papillae, retroperitoneal fibrosis, retroperitoneal tumors) Bladder outlet obstruction (e.g., prostatic hypertrophy, stones, clots, urethral strictures)
	Blocked Foley's catheter

MAJOR THREAT TO LIFE

- Renal Failure
- Hyperkalemia

Decreased urine output from any cause may result in or may be a manifestation of progressive renal insufficiency, leading to renal failure. Of the complications of renal failure, hyperkalemia is the most immediately life-threatening, as it may lead to potentially fatal cardiac dysrhythmias.

BEDSIDE

Quick Look Test

Does the patient look well (comfortable), sick (uncomfortable or distressed), or critical (about to die)?

A sick or critical looking patient suggests advanced renal insufficiency; a restless patient suggests pain from a distended bladder. However, both of these conditions can be present in a patient who appears deceptively well.

Airway and Vital Signs

Check for postural changes. A postural rise in HR > 15 beats/min, a fall in systolic BP < 15 mm Hg, or any fall in diastolic BP indicates significant hypovolemia. *Caution:* a resting tachycardia alone may indicate decreased intravascular volume.

Fever suggests concomitant urinary tract infection.

Selective Physical Examination I

Examine for *pre-renal* (volume status), *renal,* or *post-renal* (obstructive) causes of decreased urine output.

VITALS	Repeat now.
HEENT	Jaundice (hepatorenal syndrome)
	Facial purpura ⎫
	Enlarged tongue ⎬ Amyloidosis
RESP	Crackles, pleural effusions (CHF)
CVS	Pulse voume, JVP
	Skin temperature, color
ABD	Enlarged kidneys (hydronephrosis secondary to obstruction, polycystic kidney disease)
	Enlarged bladder (bladder outlet obstruction, neurogenic bladder, blocked Foley's catheter)
RECTAL	Enlarged prostate gland (bladder outlet obstruction)
PELVIC	Cervical or adnexal masses (ureteric obstruction secondary to cervical or ovarian cancer)
SKIN	Morbilliform rash (acute interstitial nephritis)
	Livedo reticularis on lower extremities (atheromatous embolic renal failure)

Selective Chart Review

Review the patient's history and hospital course, looking specifically for factors that may predispose to the pre-renal, renal, or post-renal causes of decreased urine output (see Elevator Thoughts).

Look for recent blood urea and creatinine values. A Cr/urea ratio > 12 suggests a pre-renal cause.

Management I

Your job becomes simpler when you can find a *pre-renal* or *post-renal* cause for decreased urine output.

Pre-renal

First ensure that the intravascular volume is normal. If in CHF, initiate diuresis as discussed in Chapter 20, page 207. If volume depleted, replenish the intravascular volume with NS. Add *no* potassium supplement to the IV solution until the patient passes urine. Ringer's lactate should not be given since it has potassium added to it.

Post-renal

Lower urinary tract obstruction can be adequately excluded only by passage of a Foley's catheter into the bladder.

1. If there has been bladder outlet obstruction the initial urine volume on catheterization usually will be greater than 400 ml, and the patient will experience immediate relief. Remember to listen carefully for heart murmurs before catheterizing the patient. If there is documented evidence of a cardiac valvular abnormality, SBE prophylaxis as outlined in Chapter 17, page 182, may be required. Also watch for the development of post-obstructive diuresis by monitoring urine volume status carefully for the next few days.
2. If a Foley's catheter is already in place, ensure that flushing the catheter with 20 to 30 ml of NS allows free flow of fluid from the bladder. This maneuver will exclude an intraluminal blockage of Foley's catheter as a cause of post-renal obstruction.
3. The presence of a Foley's catheter in the bladder only rules out lower urinary tract obstruction. If the preceding two steps fail to restore urine output, a *renal ultrasound* examination should be ordered first thing in the morning to exclude upper urinary tract obstruction, to document the presence of both kidneys, and to estimate renal size.

Renal

If pre-renal and post-renal factors are not operative in causing the patient's decreased urine output, you are left in the murky waters of *renal causes* of decreased urine output. A search for the renal causes of decresed urine output can wait until some more important questions are answered. (See Management II.)

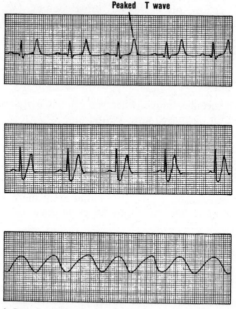

Figure 7–1. Progressive electrocardiographic features of hyperkalemia.

Management II

Regardless of the cause of decreased urine output (pre-renal, renal, or post-renal) you must now answer the following four questions:

1. **Are any of the following five life-threatening complications of decreased urine output present?**

- Hyperkalemia
- CHF
- Severe metabolic acidemia (pH < 7.2)
- Uremic encephalopathy
- Uremic pericarditis

Of these, *hyperkalemia* is the most immediately serious problem.

- Order a stat serum potassium level.
- Review the chart for a recent serum potassium level.
- Order a stat ECG if suspicion of hyperkalemia exists. Peaked T waves are early electrocardiographic signs of hyperkalemia (Fig. 7–1). More advanced ECG manifestations include depressed ST segments, prolonged PR intervals, loss of P waves, and wide QRS complexes.
- Discontinue any potassium supplements.
- Treat as outlined in Chapter 27, page 265.

Metabolic acidemia is suggested by the presence of (compensatory) hyperventilation and confirmed by ABG measurement. Investigation should take place as outlined in Appendix A, page 279.

Uremic encephalopathy manifests itself as confusion, stupor, or seizure and is managed by hemodialysis. If seizures occur they should be managed as outlined in Chapter 19 until dialysis can be initiated.

Uremic pericarditis is suggested by the presence of pleuritic chest pain, pericardial friction rub, or diffuse ST segment elevation on the ECG. It is managed best by hemodialysis.

2. **Is the patient on any drugs that may worsen the situation?**

■ Potassium supplements
■ Potassium sparing diuretics (spironolactone, triameterene, amiloride)
■ Aminoglycosides (gentamicin, netilmicin, tobramycin, amikacin)

Draw a blood sample to determine the serum level of aminoglycoside, and adjust the dosing intervals according to calculated creatinine clearance (see page 296).

3. **Is the patient in oliguric renal failure?**

If the patient has produced < 400 ml/day of urine (< 20 ml/hr), the patient has oliguric renal failure. A favor you can do for your patient is to convert this from oliguric to non-oliguric renal failure, which portends a much better prognosis.

■ Correct pre-renal and post-renal factors.
■ Give diuretics to increase urine output. *Furosemide* (Lasix) 40 mg IV given over 2 to 5 minutes. If no response, double the dose q1h (i.e., 40 to 80 to 160 mg) to a total of about 400 mg. Doses of furosemide > 100 mg should be infused at a rate not exceeding 4 mg/min to avoid ototoxicity. Smaller initial doses (e.g., 10 mg) may suffice for the patient who is frail and very elderly.
■ If furosemide is ineffective, try *ethacrynic acid* (Edecrin) 50 mg IV q60 min × 2 doses or *bumetanide* (Bumex) 1 to 10 mg IV over 1 to 2 minutes. An indwelling Foley's catheter will be required to monitor urine output in these situations.

4. **Does the patient need dialysis?**

If the patient does not pass urine despite high doses of diuretics, the indications for urgent dialysis are as follows:

■ Hyperkalemia
■ CHF
■ Metabolic acidemia (pH < 7.2)
■ Severe uremia (urea level > 35 mmol/L; creatinine level > 800 mmol/L) ± uremia seizures
■ Uremic pericarditis

If the patient is in renal failure and if one or more of these conditions is present, request an urgent nephrology consultation to dialyze the patient. While awaiting the nephrologist's arrival, all of the following problems can be temporarily treated with non-dialysis measures:

■ *Hyperkalemia:* Glucose with insulin infusion, $NaHCO_3$, calcium, sodium polystyrene sulfonate. (Refer to Chapter 27 for treatment of hyperkalemia.)
■ *CHF:* Preload measures (sit the patient up, morphine, nitroglycerin ointment). Give O_2. (Refer to Chapter 20, page 205, for management of CHF.)
■ *Metabolic acidemia:* $NaHCO_3$. (Refer to the Appendix, page 279, for assessment of metabolic acidosis.)
■ Patients with *uremic encephalopathy* should be kept calm and at bedrest until dialysis can be initiated.
■ Patients with *uremic pericarditis* may be treated symptomatically for pain with an NSAID until dialysis can be initiated.

Once these tasks have been addressed you can sit down and think about possible *renal causes* of decreased urine utput. The majority of *renal causes* are diagnosed by history, physical examination, and laboratory findings. Occasionally, a renal biopsy is required. A simple urinalysis can often provide valuable clues to the diagnosis.

■ *Urine dipstick.* Hematuria and proteinuria together suggests *glomerulonephritis.* A positive orthotoluidine test result for blood may represent hematuria, free hemoglobin, or myoglobin. Suspect *rhabdomyolysis* if there is a positive orthotoluidine test result on dipstick, but few or no RBCs on urine microscopy. (In this case, order tests of serum for CPK, Ca, and PO_4, and urine for myoglobin.)

A positive test result for urinary protein alone should prompt you to do a serum albumin and 24-hour urine collection for protein and creatinine clearance to identify the *nephrotic syndrome,* if present.

■ *Urine microscopy.* RBC casts are diagnostic of *glomerulonephritis.* Oval fat bodies are suggestive of *nephrotic syndrome.*
■ *Urine for eosinophils.* Ask for this test if there is a suspicion of *acute interstitial nephritis.*

In most cases, beyond these aforementioned simple tests, no further *investigation* is required at night.

8

FALL-OUT-OF-BED

Patients always seem to be falling out of bed—but they fall while in other places too. You will find the content of this chapter applicable to any fall occurring in the patient's room or elsewhere in the hospital.

PHONE CALL

Questions

1. **Was the fall witnessed?**
2. **Is there an obvious injury?**
3. **What are the vital signs?**
4. **Has there been a change in the level of consciousness?**
5. **Is the patient receiving anticoagulants or antiepileptic medications?**
6. **What was the reason for admission?**

Orders

Ask the RN to phone immediately if the level of consciousness changes before you are able to assess the patient.

Inform RN

"Will arrive at bedside in . . . minutes."

When other sick patients are in need of assessment, they take priority over a patient who has had an uncomplicated fall. However, a change in the level of consciousness, a fracture, or a coagulation disorder requires you to see the patient immediately.

ELEVATOR THOUGHTS (Why does a patient fall?)

CARDIAC	Dysrhythmias
	Postural hypotension (volume depletion, drugs, or autonomic failure)
	Vasovagal attack
NEURO	Confusion (in the elderly)
	Disorientation at night
	Call bell not accessible

Drugs (narcotics, sedatives, antidepressants, tranquilizers, cimetidine, antihypertensive agents)

Metabolic disorders (electrolyte abnormalities, renal failure, hepatic failure)

Dementia (Parkinson's disease, Alzheimer's disease, multi-infarction)

TIA, stroke

Seizure

ENVIRONMENTAL   There are many potential environmental hazards within the hospital setting, e.g., a fall on a wet floor, a fall during an unassisted transfer from bed to chair, and a fall while walking in a patient who requires assistance.

MAJOR THREAT TO LIFE

Head Injury

Any patient who may have hit his or her head during a fall requires a complete neurologic examination now. Even seemingly minor trauma can result in a serious intracranial bleed in an anticoagulated patient. If a new neurologic problem is identified, an immediate CT scan of the head can be helpful. The consideration of immediate reversal of anticoagulation should be discussed in consultation with your resident and hematologist. (See Chapter 25, page 255 for reversal of anticoagulation.) If no neurologic deficit is identified at this time, observation by frequent assessment of the neuro-vital signs is required.

BEDSIDE

Quick Look Test

Does the patient look well (comfortable), sick (uncomfortable or distressed), or critical (about to die)?

Most patients do not have life-threatening problems to account for falling. Usually they look well, and the vital signs are normal.

Airway and Vital Signs

What is the heart rate and rhythm?

A tachycardia, bradycardia, or an irregular rhythm may indicate a dysrhythmia as the cause of the fall.

Are there postural (lying and sitting) changes in BP and HR?

If there are postural changes, recheck the BP and HR with the patient standing. A postural fall in BP together with a postural rise in HR (> 15 beats/min) suggests volume depletion. A drop in BP without a change in HR suggests autonomic dysfunction. An initial drop in BP that corrects on standing also suggests autonomic dysfunction. Drugs are common causes of postural hypotension in elderly patients.

Selective History

Ask the patient why he or she fell—after all, they may know the answer!
Is the patient aware of any injury sustained during the fall?
Patients may fracture a hip as a result of falling. However, it is not uncommon for an elderly patient to sustain a fracture of the femoral neck while walking and subsequently fall.

Were there any warning symptoms prior to the fall?
Lightheadedness and visual disturbances on standing may indicate postural hypotension. Palpitations suggest a dysrhythmia. Auras are rare but, if present, are highly suggestive of a seizure disorder.

What was the patient doing just prior to the fall?
Coughing, micturating, or straining are examples of maneuvers that may result in vasovagal syncope.

Is there a history of previous falls?
Recurrent falls suggest an underlying disorder that has gone unrecognized. Here is your chance to shine!

Is the patient diabetic?
Hyperglycemia or hypoglycemia may cause confusion, and the patient may, as a consequence, fall. Order a chemstrip or glucometer reading. Check the diabetic record for the past 3 days.

Question any witnesses who observed the fall.

Selective Physical Examination

VITALS	Repeat now. Only supine BP and HR are necessary, provided both supine and standing measurements were already taken.
HEENT	Tongue or cheek lacerations (seizure)
	Hemotympanum (basal skull fracture)
CVS	Pulse rate and rhythm (dysrhythmia)
	Decreased JVP (volume depletion)

MSS   Palpate skull and face   ⎫
           Palpate spine and ribs   ⎬ Fractures, hematomas,
           Passive ROM of all four   ⎭ lacerations
              limbs
NEURO   Complete neurologic examination. Pay particular at-
           tention to the level of consciousness and to any
           asymmetric neurologic findings. New findings of
           asymmetry suggest structural brain disease.

Selective Chart Review (Search for the cause of the fall.)

1. **What was the reason for admission?**
2. **Is there a past history of cardiac dysrhythmia, seizure disorder, autonomic neuropathy, disorientation at night, or diabetes mellitus?**
3. **Which drugs is the patient receiving?**

- Antihypertensives
- Diuretics (volume depletion)
- Antidysrhythmics
- Antiepileptics
- Narcotics
- Sedatives, tranquilizers
- Antidepressants
- Insulin, oral hypoglycemics

4. **Check the most recent laboratory results.**

- Glucose ⎫
- Na   ⎬ ↑ or ↓ may cause confusion.
- ↑ K can cause AV blocks; ↓ K can cause weakness or PVCs.
- ↑ Ca causes confusion; ↓ Ca causes seizures.
- Urea, creatinine (Uremia can result in confusion and seizures.)
- Antiepileptic drug concentrations (Sub-therapeutic concentrations may result in seizure breakthrough; toxic concentrations may be associated with ataxia.)

Management

Provisional Diagnosis. Establish the reason for the fall (*provisional diagnosis*). The etiology is often multifactorial. For example, diuretic-induced nocturia forces an elderly patient, under the influence of nighttime sedation, to struggle to the bathroom in an unfamiliar, dimly lit hospital room.

Complications. Are there any *complications* resulting from the fall, giving rise to a second diagnosis?

For example, the stroke victim may have unknowingly dislocated or subluxated his or her shoulder on the paralyzed side during the fall. The anticoagulated patient may develop a serious, delayed hemorrhage at any site of trauma. Re-examine these patients frequently.

Treat the Cause. Investigate and *treat the suspected cause*. A fall is a symptom, not a diagnosis!

Reversible Factors. Reversible factors must be corrected, especially volume depletion and inappropriate drug therapy in the elderly.

Nocturia. The majority of elderly patients who fall-out-of-bed at night are on their way to the bathroom because of nocturia. Make sure the nocturia is not iatrogenic (e.g., an evening diuretic order or an unnecessary IV)!

Elderly Patient. If the elderly patient is disoriented at night, ensure that the side rails are left up, the call bell is easily accessible, a night light is left on, and the evening's fluid intake is limited.

9

FEVER

It is unusual to spend an entire night on-call without being phoned about a febrile patient. The majority of fevers seen in hospitalized patients are due to infections. Locating the source of a fever usually requires some detective work. Whether the cause of the fever needs specific immediate treatment will depend both on the clinical status of the patient and on the suspected diagnosis.

PHONE CALL

Questions

1. **How high is the temperature and by what route was it taken?**
   37°C oral = 37.5°C rectal or 36.5°C axillary
2. **What are the other vital signs?**
3. **Are there any associated symptoms?**
   Ask specifically about headache, seizure, and change in sensorium—each of which may indicate possible meningitis. Other symptoms may help you localize the site of infection. Rigors (shaking chills) in a patient in the hospital suggest bacteremia.
4. **Is this a "new" fever?**
5. **What was the reason for admission?**
6. **Is this a post-operative patient?**
   Fever occurring 24 to 48 hours after an operation is usually due to atelectasis; fever occurring 5 days after an operation is usually due to pneumonia; and fever occurring 10 days after an operation is suggestive of pulmonary embolism.

Orders

1. If febrile and hypotensive, give IV 500 ml NS as rapidly as possible.
2. If febrile with "meningitis symptoms," order an LP tray to the bedside now.

Inform RN

"Will arrive at bedside in . . . minutes."

An elevated temperature alone is seldom life-threatening. However, fever in association with hypotension or "meningitis symptoms" requires you to see the patient immediately.

ELEVATOR THOUGHTS (What causes fever?)

1. *Infection* is by far the most common cause of fever in the hospitalized patient. Common sites of infection are the lung and urinary tract. Less common sites include skin (IV sites), CNS, abdomen, and pelvis.
2. Post-operative atelectasis
3. Pulmonary embolism
4. Drug-induced fever
5. Neoplasm
6. Connective tissue diseases

MAJOR THREAT TO LIFE

■ Septic shock
■ Meningitis

Fever is most commonly a manifestation of infection in the hospitalized patient. Most infections can be brought under control by a combination of the body's natural defense mechanisms and judicious antibiotic use. *Meningitis,* by virtue of its location, can result in permanent neurologic deficit or death, if allowed to go untreated. Infection at any site, if progressive, may lead to septicemia with attendant *septic shock.*

BEDSIDE

Quick Look Test

Does the patient look well (comfortable), sick (uncomfortable or distressed), or critical (about to die)?
"Toxic signs," such as apprehension, agitation, and lethargy, suggest serious infection.

Airway and Vital Signs

What is the heart rate?
Tachycardia, proportionate to the temperature elevation, is an expected finding in the febrile patient. A relative bradycardia in the febrile patient is said to occur in *Legionella* pneumonia, ascending cholangitis, and typhoid fever.

What is the blood pressure?
Fever in association with supine or postural hypotension indicates relative hypovolemia and can be the forerunner of septic shock. Ensure that an IV is in place. Infuse NS or Ringer's lactate to correct the intravascular volume deficit.

Selective Physical Examination I

What is the volume status? Is the patient in septic shock? Are there signs of meningitis?

VITALS	Repeat now.
HEENT	Photophobia, neck stiffness
CVS	Pulse volume, JVP, skin temperature and color
NEURO	Change in sensorium
SPECIAL	
MANEUVERS	*Brudzinski's sign:* With the patient supine, passively flex the neck forward. Flexion of the patient's hips and knees in response to this maneuver constitutes a positive test result (see Chapter 11, Fig. 11–3A).
	Kernig's sign: With the patient supine, flex one hip and knee to 90 degrees, then straighten the knee. Pain or resistance in the ipsilateral hamstrings constitutes a positive test result (see Chapter 11, Fig. 11–3B).

Septic shock is a clinical diagnosis consisting of two stages. Serious delays in treatment are made through failure to recognize the first stage. Early in the development of septic shock, the patient may be warm, dry, and flushed because of peripheral vasodilation and increased cardiac output ("warm shock"). As septic shock progresses, the patient becomes cool, clammy, and hypotensive ("cold shock"), owing to peripheral vasoconstriction.

Fever in the elderly patient, regardless of cause, can produce changes in sensorium ranging from lethargy to agitation. If a specific site of infection is not obvious, an LP should be performed to rule out meningitis (see page 69).

Management I

What immediate measures need to be taken to prevent septic shock or to recognize meningitis?

Septic Shock

If the patient is febrile and hypotensive, determine the volume status and give IV fluids (NS or Ringer's lactate) promptly until the volume status returns to normal. Aggressive volume repletion in a patient with a history of CHF may compromise cardiac function. Do not overshoot the mark!

While IV fluid resuscitation is taking place, obtain samples for necessary cultures, usually including blood from two different sites, urine (for Gram's stain and culture), and any other potentially infected body fluid.

Septic shock is a major threat to life, and once culture samples are taken, antibiotics must be given to cover both gram-positive and gram-negative organisms. A common, empiric broad-spectrum regimen includes a cephalosporin and an aminoglycoside, e.g., *cefazolin* (Ancef) 1 to 2 gm IV q8hr and *gentamicin* 2 to 3 mg/kg IV as a loading dose. Further maintenance doses of gentamicin should be 1.5 mg/kg IV given at an interval that is adjusted for creatinine clearance.

Many patients are allergic to penicillin. Ensure that the patient is *not* allergic before ordering penicillin or cephalosporin.

Aminoglycosides are common causes of nephrotoxicity and oto-toxicity. Select maintenance dosing intervals according to the patient's calculated CrCl (see Appendix, page 296). Follow the serum aminoglycoside concentrations, usually after the third or fourth dose, and the serum creatinine concentration.

If the volume status is normal and the patient is still hypotensive, transfer to the ICU/CCU for inotropic or vasopressor support. (Refer to Chapter 15 for further discussion of septic shock.)

A Foley's catheter should be placed in a patient with a case of septic shock to monitor urine output.

Meningitis

Signs of Meningitis

Fever plus headache, seizure, stiff neck, or change in sensorium is *meningitis* until proved otherwise.

If, on fundoscopic examination, there is no evidence of raised intracranial pressure (see Chapter 11, Fig. 11–2) and if a CT scan of the head is not immediately available, perform an LP without delay. If you are unable to visualize the fundi or if there is papilledema, give the first dose of antibiotics and arrange for an urgent CT scan of the head to exclude a space-occupying lesion before performing the LP.

An LP done in the presence of an intracranial space-occupying lesion can result in uncal herniation and brain stem compression ("coning").

Selective Chart Review

If the patient is not in septic shock and does not have symptoms or signs of meningitis perform a selective chart review—looking for *localizing clues* (Table 9–1). Also check the chart for the following:

- Temperature pattern during hospital stay
- Recent WBC count and differential
- Allergies to antibiotics
- Other possible reasons for fever, e.g., connective tissue disease, neoplasm
- Antipyretics, antibiotics, or steroids that may modify the fever pattern.

Table 9–1. SELECTIVE CHART REVIEW—LOOKING FOR LOCALIZING CLUES

Localizing Clues	Diagnostic Considerations	Comments
Recent surgery	Atelectasis	Post-operative fever due to atelectasis is a diagnosis to be made after exclusion of infection.
	Pneumonia	Characteristically presents 5 days post-operatively.
	Pulmonary embolism	Characteristically presents 7 to 10 days post-operatively.
	Infected surgical wound, biopsy site, or deeper infection of biopsy organ	Despite modern surgical techniques, *any* incision or puncture site may serve as a portal for bacteria.
Blood transfusion	Transfusion reaction	See Chapter 23
Headache, seizure, stiff neck, changes in sensorium	Meningitis Intracranial abscess Encephalitis	Delirium tremens can mimic meningitis in some patients. Is the patient withdrawing from alcohol?
Sinus discomfort	Sinusitis	
Dental caries, toothache	Periodontal abscess	
Sore throat	Pharyngitis Tonsillitis	
Dysphagia	Retropharyngeal abscess Epiglottitis	Either of these diagnoses is a medical emergency. Consult ENT or anesthesia immediately.
SOB, cough, or chest pain	Pneumonia Lung abscess Pulmonary embolus	
Murmur, CHF, or peripheral embolic lesions	Infectious endocarditis	
Pleuritic chest pain	Pneumonia Empyema Pulmonary embolus Pericarditis	
Costovertebral angle (CVA) tenderness	Pyelonephritis Perinephric abscess	
Foley's catheter, dysuria, hematuria, or pyuria	Cystitis Pyelonephritis	Both condom catheters and Foley's catheters predispose patients to urinary tract infections.
Abdominal pain RUQ	Subphrenic abscess Hepatic abscess Hepatitis RLL pneumonia Ascending cholangitis	If there are peritoneal signs, consider surgical consultation. Does the patient have Charcot's triad (fever + RUQ pain + jaundice)? If so, consider surgical consultation.
RLQ	Crohn's disease Appendicitis Salpingitis	

Table 9–1. SELECTIVE CHART REVIEW—LOOKING FOR LOCALIZING CLUES *Continued*

Localizing Clues	Diagnostic Considerations	Comments
LUQ	Splenic abscess	
	Infected pancreatic pseudocyst	
	LLL pneumonia	
LLQ	Diverticular abscess	
	Salpingitis	
Ascites	Peritonitis	Perform abdominal paracentesis to exclude spontaneous bacterial peritonitis in any ascitic patient who becomes unwell.
Diarrhea	Enteritis	
	Colitis	
Swollen red tender joint	Septic arthritis	A monoarticular effusion *must* be tapped to exclude infection.
	Gout or pseudogout	
Prosthetic joint	Infected prosthesis	
Vaginal discharge	Endometritis	
	Salpingitis	
Red or tender IV site	Septic phlebitis	
TPN line	Catheter sepsis	Fever may be the only symptom.

Selective Physical Examination II

Confirm localizing symptoms or signs already documented in chart review.

VITALS   Repeat now.

HEENT   Fundi—papilledema (intracranial abscess); Roth's spots (infective endocarditis) (Fig. 9–1)

        Conjunctival or scleral petechiae (infectious endocarditis)

        Ears—red tympanic membranes (otitis media, a complication of the intubated patient)

        Sinuses—tenderness, inability to transilluminate (sinusitis)

        Oral cavity—dental caries, tender tooth on palpation (periodontal abscess)

        Pharynx—erythema, pharyngeal exudate (pharyngitis)

        Neck—stiff (meningitis)

RESP   Crackles, friction rub, signs of consolidation (pneumonia, pulmonary embolism)

CVS   New murmurs (infectious endocarditis)

ABD   Localized tenderness (see page 25)

RECTAL   Tenderness or mass (rectal abscess)

MSS   Joint erythema or effusion (septic arthritis)

SKIN   Decubitus ulcers (cellulitis)

       Osler's nodes and Janeway's lesions (Fig. 9–2)

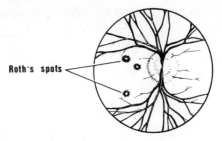

Figure 9–1. Roth's spots. Round or oval hemorrhagic retinal lesions with central pallor.

Petechiae (infectious endocarditis)
IV sites (phlebitis, cellulitis)

PELVIC   A pelvic examination should be done if a pelvic source of fever is possible.

Management II

Any patient with an unexplained oral temperature > 38.5°C should have the following:

- Blood cultures immediately from two different sites
- Urinalysis (routine and microscopic) and urine culture immediately
- WBC count and differential

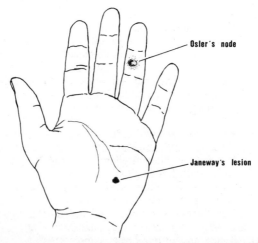

Figure 9–2. Osler's node. Tender nodules, 2 to 5 mm in diameter, found in the tips of the digits. Janeway's lesion. Non-tender erythematous macules on the palms and soles.

Other more *selective tests* depend upon the *localizing clues* you have been able to elicit with your chart review, history, and physical examination.

- Throat swab for Gram's stain and culture
- CXR
- LP
- Blood cultures for infectious endocarditis (refer to your institution's protocol).
- Cervical culture (also obtain specific medium for gonococcal isolation prior to performing the pelvic examination).
- Joint aspiration
- Swab decubitus ulcers for Gram's stain and culture.
- Retrograde milking of IV sites for purulent exudate for Gram's stain and culture

Fluid from any source should be examined microscopically, immediately to help in your choice of antibiotics.

Remove *suspected IVs* and replace if necessary at a new site. Central TPN lines that may be infected should be replaced in consultation with your resident or TPN service. Catheter tips should be sent to the laboratory for culture.

Remove a Foley's catheter in a patient suspected of having *urinary tract infection*. A few days of incontinence in the patient is an annoyance for the nursing staff but will not harm the patient, if there is no perineal skin breakdown. An exception to this occurs when a Foley's catheter is placed to treat urinary retention, since urinary stasis predisposes the patient to infection.

In regard to *antibiotic selection*, which patient needs *broad-spectrum antibiotics* now?

The patient with *fever and hypotension* requires broad-spectrum antibiotics (see page 69).

The patient (e.g., on chemotherapy) with *fever and neutropenia* ($< 500/mm^3$) may not have enough WBCs to produce the localizing signs seen in an immunocompetent host. A minimum workup includes the following:

- Urinalysis and urine culture
- Sputum for Gram's stain and culture
- CXR

Anticipate this event and agree upon an appropriate broad-spectrum antibiotic regimen with the hematologist or oncologist well ahead of time.

Which patient needs *specific antibiotics* now?

The patient with *fever and meningitis symptoms* requires antibiotics immediately after the LP is done. However, do not delay initial antibiotic treatment if a CT scan of the head must be done before the LP (see page 69).

The patient with *fever and a clear localizing clue* should be given specific antibiotics following procurement of culture specimens. Antibiotic therapy should be considered an urgent requirement in the diabetic patient.

Which patient needs *no antibiotics* until a specific microbiologic diagnosis is made?

A patient who does not look sick or critical and in whom the source of fever is not readily apparent (e.g., a patient admitted for workup of FUO).

Low grade fever ($< 38.5°C$) in a patient who doesn't look sick.

Which antibiotics should you choose?

The common infecting organisms change much more slowly than the antibiotics synthesized to inhibit them! Specific antibiotic choices depend upon knowledge of your hospital's local microbial flora and their antibiotic sensitivities. Current guidelines may be found in Appendix B, page 298.

REMEMBER

1. The definition of FUO is a temperature $>38.3°C$ for 3 weeks with no cause found despite thorough in-hospital investigation for 1 week.
2. Fever due to neoplasm, connective tissue disorder, or drug reaction is a diagnosis to be made *after* exclusion of fever due to infection.
3. Drug-induced fever is rare and usually occurs within 7 days of beginning the offending drug.
4. Treating a fever with antipyretics is only treating a symptom. It is useful to observe the fever pattern, and, if the patient is not uncomfortable, it is not necessary to treat with aspirin or acetaminophen.
5. If antipyretics are ordered, ask the RN to indicate with an arrow the time of administration on the bedside temperature chart. In addition, assessment of therapeutic response is made easier by charting the antibiotics given as well (Fig. 9–3).
6. Steroids may elevate the WBC count and suppress fever response, regardless of the cause. Defervescence with steroids should be interpreted cautiously.
7. Microorganisms love foreign bodies. Look for foreign bodies as sites of infection—IVs, Foley's catheters, VP shunts, prosthetic joints, peritoneal dialysis catheters, and porcine or mechanical heart valves.
8. Fevers occurring while the patient is already on antibiotics may mean the following:
   (a) You are not giving the right dose.

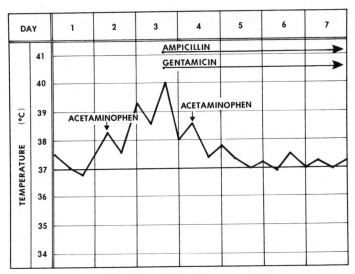

Figure 9–3. Bedside temperature chart.

(b) You are not treating the right organism or resistance or superinfection has developed.

(c) The antibiotic is not getting to the right place (e.g., thick-walled abscess).

(d) The fever may not be due to an infection.

9. Delirium tremens is a serious cause of fever occasionally seen in patients withdrawing from alcohol. It is associated with confusion, including delusions and hallucinations, agitation, seizures, and signs of autonomic hyperactivity, including fever, tachycardia, and sweating. This condition is often fatal and requires high doses of benzodiazepines to stabilize the patient (see page 48).

10

GASTROINTESTINAL BLEEDING

GI bleeding is common in hospitalized patients. Whether the bleeding is from minor gastric stress ulceration or from life-threatening exsanguination of aortoduodenal fistula, the initial principles of assessment and management are the same.

PHONE CALL

Questions

1. Clarify the situation. **(Is the blood old or new and from where is it coming?)**
   Vomiting of bright red blood or "coffee grounds" and most cases of melena indicate an upper GI bleed. Bright red blood passed rectally usually indicates a lower GI bleed.
2. **How much blood has been lost?**
3. **What are the vital signs?**
   This information helps determine the urgency of the situation.
4. **What was the admitting diagnosis?**
   Recurrent bleeding from duodenal ulcer or esophageal varices carries a high mortality rate.
5. **Is the patient receiving anticoagulants (heparin, warfarin)?**
   Anticoagulation will require immediate discontinuation or reversal in an actively bleeding patient.

Orders

1. Large bore IV (size 16 if possible) immediately, if not already in place. IV access is a priority in the bleeding patient.
2. Hb stat. *Caution:* The Hb level may be normal during an acute bleed and drops only with correction of the intravascular volume by a shift of fluid from the extravascular space.
3. Crossmatch: Is there blood on hold? If not, order stat crossmatch for 2, 4, or 6 units of packed RBCs, depending on your estimate of blood loss.
4. If the admitting diagnosis is bleeding esophageal varices and the patient is hypotensive, order a Minnesota (Sengstaken-Blakemore) tube to be at the bedside immediately. If not familiar with the use of this tube call your resident for assistance now.
5. Ask the RN to take the patient's chart to the bedside.

Inform RN

"Will arrive at bedside in . . . minutes."

Hypotension or tachycardia requires you to see the patient immediately.

ELEVATOR THOUGHTS (What causes GI bleeds?)

Upper GI Bleed

1. Esophagitis
2. Esophageal varices
3. Mallory-Weiss syndrome (tear)
4. Gastritis
5. Gastric ulcer
6. Duodenitis
7. Duodenal ulcer

Lower GI Bleed

1. Neoplasm
2. Angiodysplasia
3. Diverticulosis
4. Ischemic colitis
5. Mesenteric thrombosis
6. Meckel's diverticulum
7. Hemorrhoids

MAJOR THREAT TO LIFE

Hypovolemic Shock

The major concern with GI bleeding is the progressive loss of intravascular volume in the patient whose bleeding lesion is not identified and managed correctly. If allowed to progress, even minor intermittent or continuous bleeding may eventually result in hypovolemic shock with hypoperfusion of vital organs.

Initially, lost blood volume may be corrected by infusion of NS or Ringer's lactate, but if bleeding continues replacement of lost RBCs will also be required in the form of packed RBC transfusions. Hence, your initial assessment should be directed towards determining the patient's volume status to ascertain whether a significant amount of intravascular volume has been lost.

BEDSIDE

Quick Look Test

Does the patient look well (comfortable), sick (uncomfortable or distressed), or critical (about to die)?

The patient in hypovolemic shock due to blood loss appears pale and apprehensive and may have other symptoms and signs, including cold and clammy skin, due to stimulation of the sympathetic nervous system.

Airway and Vital Signs

Are there postural changes in blood pressure or heart rate?

First check for changes with the patient in the lying and sitting positions. If there are no changes, the BP and HR should then be checked with the patient standing. A rise in heart rate > 15 beats/min, a fall in systolic BP > 15 mm Hg, or fall in diastolic BP indicates significant hypovolemia. *Caution:* A resting tachycardia alone may indicate decreased intravascular volume.

If the resting systolic BP is < 90 mm Hg, order a second large bore IV immediately.

Selective Physical Examination I

What is the patient's volume status? Is the patient in shock?

VITALS	Repeat now.
CVS	Pulse volume, JVP
	Skin temperature and color
NEURO	Mental status

Shock is a clinical diagnosis as follows: systolic BP < 90 mm Hg with evidence of inadequate tissue perfusion, e.g., skin (cold and clammy) and CNS (agitation or confusion). In fact, the kidney is a sensitive indicator of shock (i.e., urine output < 20 ml/hr). The urine output of a patient who is hypovolemic ordinarily correlates with the renal blood flow which, in turn, is dependent on cardiac output and is an extremely important measurement. However, placement of a Foley's catheter should not take priority over resuscitation measures.

Management

What immediate measures need to be taken to correct or prevent shock from occurring?

Replenish the intravascular volume by giving IV fluids. The best immediate choice is a crystalloid (NS or Ringer's lactate), which will at least temporarily stay in the intravascular space. Albumin or banked plasma can be given but is expensive, carries a risk of hepatitis, and is not readily available.

Blood has been lost from the intravascular space, and ideally blood is what needs to be replaced. If there is no blood on hold for the patient, a stat crossmatch will usually take 50 minutes. If blood is on hold, it should be available at the bedside in 30 minutes. In an emergency, O-negative blood may be given, though this practice is usually reserved for the acute trauma victim. Transfusion-associated hepatitis can be minimized by transfusing only when necessary. Rule-of-thumb: Maintain a Hb level of 90 to 100 g/L.

Order the appropriate IV rate, which will depend upon the patient's volume status. *Shock* will require running IV fluid "wide open" through at least two large bore IV sites. Elevating the IV bag, squeezing the IV bag, or using IV pressure cuffs may help increase the rate of delivery of the solution. *Moderate volume depletion* can be treated with 500 to 1000 ml of NS given as rapidly as possible with serial measurements of volume status and assessment of cardiac status. If blood is not at the bedside within 30 minutes, delegate someone to find out why there is a delay. Aggressive volume repletion in a patient with a history of CHF may compromise cardiac function. Do not overshoot the mark!

What can you do at this time to stop the source of bleeding?

Treat the underlying cause. Treating hypovolemia is treating a symptom.

Upper GI Bleed (Hematemesis and Most Cases of Melena). *Cimetidine* (Tagamet) 300 mg IV q6h (300 mg IV q12h in renal failure) or *ranitidine* (Zantac) 50 mg IV q8h (50 mg IV q12h in renal failure) will help promote healing in five of the seven causes listed (i.e., all except Mallory-Weiss syndrome (tear) and esophageal varices). Studies have failed to show the H_2 blockers decrease the incidence of rebleeding while patients are in the hospital. Most specialists still would begin one, until the specific site of bleeding is known. Antacids are contraindicated if endoscopy or surgery is anticipated. They obscure the field in endoscopy and increase the risk of aspiration in surgery.

Lower GI Bleed (Usually Bright Red Blood per Rectum and, occasionally, Melena). No other treatment is immediately required until specific site of bleeding is identified but continue to monitor the volume status.

Abnormal Coagulation. If the PT or aPTT are prolonged and if the patient is thrombocytopenic, fresh frozen plasma (2 units) and platelet infusion (6 to 8 units), respectively, may be required.

Selective Chart Review

What was the reason for admission?

Has the cause for this GI bleed already been identified during this admission?

Is the patient on any medication that may worsen the situation?

KCl	Irritates gastric mucosa.
NSAIDs	Counteract the protective effect of prostaglandins on gastric mucosa and may increase bleeding time.
Steroids	Increased frequency of ulcer disease in patients on steroids. Most disease processes for which the patient is receiving steroids will not allow their immediate discontinuation.
Heparin	Prevents clot formation by enhancing the action of antithrombin III.
Warfarin	Prevents activation of vitamin K–dependent clotting factors.

Laboratory Data

- Most recent Hb value
- PT, aPTT, platelets. Are there any platelet or coagulation abnormalities that may predispose the patient to bleeding?
- Bleeding time
- Urea, creatinine levels. (Uremia prolongs bleeding time.) Remember, in prerenal failure urea level may be more markedly elevated than creatinine level. This difference may be further accentuated in a GI bleed by absorption of urea from the breakdown of blood in the GI tract.

Selective Physical Examination II

Where is the site of bleeding?

VITALS	Repeat now.
HEENT	Nosebleed
CVS	JVP, atrial fibrillation (mesenteric embolus)
ABD	Epigastric tenderness (peptic ulcer disease)
	RLQ tenderness or mass (cecal cancer)
	LLQ tenderness (sigmoid cancer, diverticulitis, or ischemic colitis)
RECTAL	Bright red blood, melena, hemorrhoids, or mass (rectal cancer)

Also, look for signs of chronic liver disease (parotid gland hypertrophy, spider angiomata, gynecomastia, palmar erythema, testicular atrophy, dilated abdominal veins), which may suggest the presence of esophageal varices.

Management II

Does the *specific site of bleeding* need to be established now?
No—first correct hypovolemia.

What *procedures* are available to determine the site of bleeding?

- Esophagogastroduodenoscopy
- Tagged RBC scan
- Angiography
- Sigmoidoscopy
- Colonoscopy

In a patient with an upper GI bleed that has stopped and who is stable hemodynamically, elective endoscopy can be performed within the next 24 hours. An angiography or a tagged RBC scan is most sensitive if performed while there is still active bleeding, but should not take priority over resuscitation measures.

When is *early surgical consultation* appropriate?

- Exsanguinating hemorrhage
- Continued bleeding with transfusion requirements > 5 units/day
- A second bleed from an ulcer, requiring transfusion during the same hospital stay
- Ulcer with a visible vessel at the base on endoscopy

Order an ECG and cardiac enzyme tests if there are any risk factors for coronary artery disease. A hypotensive episode in a patient with atherosclerosis may result in myocardial infarction.

Esophageal varices can be treated with sclerotherapy, a vasopressin infusion (100 units in 250 ml D5W beginning at a rate of 0.3 units/min = 45 ml/hr), or a Minnesota (Sengstaken-Blakemore) tube (Fig. 10–1). In most cases the presence of bleeding varices should be documented endoscopically before initiating any treatment. Sclerotherapy is the preferred elective treatment, as vasopressin may precipitate angina or MI in the atherosclerotic patient. A Minnesota tube is a temporizing measure reserved for a life-threatening bleed.

REMEMBER

1. Keep the patient NPO for endoscopy or possible surgery.
2. Insertion of an NG tube to look for bright red blood may help identify an UGI source of bleeding. However, negative NG returns do not rule out an UGI bleed. Do not leave the NG tube in to monitor bleeding. The patient's volume status is the best indicator of further blood loss, and an NG tube may cause mucosal artifacts, hampering interpretation of endoscopic findings.
3. Bismuth compounds (e.g., Pepto-Bismol) and iron supplements can turn stools black. True melena is pitch black, sticky, and tar-like, with an odor that is hard to forget.

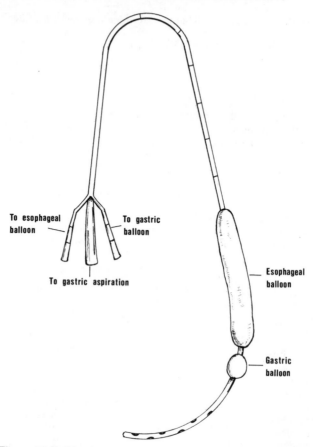

Figure 10–1. The Sengstaken-Blakemore tube. The Minnesota tube is similar; it has an additional port for esophageal aspiration.

4. An aortoduodenal fistula can appear as a sentinel (minor) bleed which can then be followed by rapid exsanguination. Consider this possibility in any patient with abdominal vascular surgery or in any patient with a midline abdominal scar who is unable to give a history.
5. Never attribute a GI bleed to hemorrhoids before thorough exclusion of other sources of bleeding.

11

HEADACHE

Chronic headaches are common problems. Patients in the hospital often complain of headaches. You must decide whether the headache is chronic and of no urgent concern or whether it is a symptom of more serious concern.

PHONE CALL

Questions

1. **How severe is the headache?**
   Most headaches are mild and not of major concern unless associated with other symptoms.
2. **Was the onset sudden or gradual?**
   The sudden onset of a severe headache is suggestive of a subarachnoid hemorrhage.
3. **What are the vital signs?**
4. **Has there been a change in the level of consciousness?**
5. **Is there a past history of chronic or recurrent headaches?**
6. **What was the reason for admission?**

Orders

1. Ask the RN to measure the patient's temperature, if it has not been recorded within the past hour. Bacterial meningitis may be present with only fever and headache.
2. If you are confident that the headache represents a chronic or previously diagnosed, recurrent problem, the patient can be given medication that has previously relieved the headache or a non-narcotic analgesic agent (acetaminophen). Ask the RN to phone back in 2 hours if the headache is not relieved by the medication.

Inform RN

"Will arrive at the bedside in . . . minutes."
Headaches associated with a fever or a decreased level of consciousness and severe headaches of acute onset require you to see the patient immediately. Assessment, at the bedside, of chronic or recurrent headaches is necessary if there is concern that the headache is more severe than usual or if the character of the pain

is different. This assessment can wait an hour or two if other problems of higher priority exist.

ELEVATOR THOUGHTS (What causes headaches?)

Chronic (Recurrent) Headaches

1. Psychogenic
   "Tension headache"
   Depression
   Anxiety
2. Vascular
   Migraine
   Cluster

Acute Headaches

1. Infectious
   Meningitis
   Encephalitis
2. Post-trauma
   Concussion
   Subdural or epidural hematoma
3. Vascular
   Subarachnoid hemorrhage
   Intracerebral hemorrhage
4. Increased intracranial pressure
   Space-occupying lesions
   Malignant hypertension
   Benign intracranial hypertension
5. Local causes
   Temporal arteritis
   Acute angle–closure glaucoma

MAJOR THREAT TO LIFE

- Bacterial meningitis
- Herniation (transtentorial, cerebellar, central)

Bacterial meningitis must be recognized early if antibiotic treatment is to be successful. Herniation may occur as a result of a tumor, subdural or epidural hematoma, or any other mass lesion (Fig. 11–1).

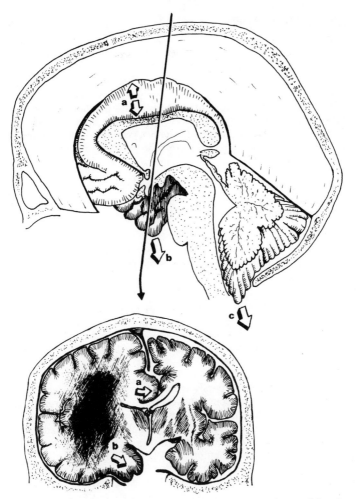

Figure 11–1. CNS herniation. a. cingulate herniation, b. uncal herniation, and c. cerebellar herniation.

BEDSIDE

Quick Look Test

Does the patient look well (comfortable), sick (uncomfortable or distressed), or critical (about to die)?

Most patients with chronic headaches look well. Those with severe migraines look sick.

Airway and Vital Signs

What is the temperature?

Fever associated with a headache requires you to decide soon whether an LP should be done.

What is the BP?

Malignant hypertension (hypertension with papilledema) is usually associated with a systolic BP > 190 mm Hg and a diastolic BP > 120 mm Hg. Headache is not usually a symptom of hypertension unless there has been a recent increase in pressure, and the diastolic BP is > 120 mm Hg.

What is the HR?

Hypertension in association with bradycardia may be a manifestation of increasing intracranial pressure.

Selective Physical Examination I (Does the patient have meningitis or increased intracranial pressure?)

HEENT   Nuchal rigidity (meningitis or subarachnoid hemorrhage)

Papilledema (increased intracranial pressure)

An early sign of increased intracranial pressure is absence of venous pulsations. See Figure 11–2 for the fundoscopic features of papilledema.

NEURO   Mental status

Pupil symmetry

Asymmetric pupils associated with a rapidly decreasing level of consciousness represent a life-threatening situation. Call neurosurgery immediately for assessment and treatment of probable uncal herniation.

Kernig's sign and Brudzinski's sign (meningitis or subarachnoid hemorrhage) (Fig. 11–3).

A full neurologic examination is required, if there is nuchal rigidity or pupillary asymmetry.

Management I

If there is *nuchal rigidity without papilledema* order

Immediate CT scan of the head

LP tray

Note the time. If bacterial meningitis is suspected, you should be able to complete the CT scan of the head followed by the LP with the patient receiving the first IV dose of antibiotics within 1 hour.

When bacterial meningitis is suspected, but the CT scan of the

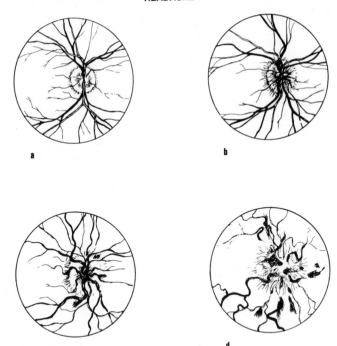

Figure 11–2. Disc changes seen in papilledema. a = normal, b = early papilledema, c = moderate papilledema with early hemorrhage, and d = severe papilledema with extensive hemorrhage.

head is not available within the hour, utilize one of two alternatives as follows: (1) perform an LP to be followed by IV antibiotics and (2) give appropriate, empiric IV antibiotics now (see subsequent discussion), performing an LP after the CT scan of the head is available.

If there is *nuchal rigidity with papilledema,* an LP is contraindicated because of the risk of brain herniation.

Meningitis, a subdural empyema, and a brain abscess can each appear with nuchal rigidity and papilledema. The CT scan of the head may help differentiate among the three. The empiric antibiotic coverage is as follows:

Bacterial Meningitis

Adult   Penicillin G 2 million units IV over 30 min-
                          utes q2h or 4 million units IV q4h

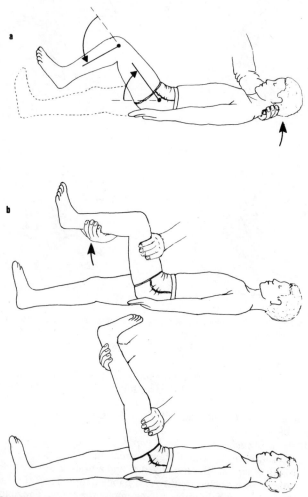

Figure 11–3. a = Brudzinski's sign. The test result is positive when the patient actively flexes his or her hips and knees in response to passive neck flexion by the examiner. b = Kernig's sign. The test result is positive when pain or resistance is elicited by passive knee extension, from the 90-degree hip/knee flexion position.

Immunosuppressed, Alcoholic, or > 60 years	A third generation cephalosporin that crosses the blood-brain barrier plus an aminoglycoside
Post-craniotomy, Spinal Trauma (Within the First 3 Days)	Penicillin G 10 million units/day IV
Post-craniotomy, Spinal Trauma (After the First 3 Days)	A third generation cephalosporin that crosses the blood-brain barrier plus an aminoglycoside plus a penicillinase-resistant penicillin

Subdural Empyema and Brain Abscess

Secondary to Frontoethmoid Sinusitis	Penicillin G 15 to 20 million units/day IV plus nafcillin 10 to 15 gm/day plus chloramphenicol 4 gm/day (60 to 90% of subdural empyemas are caused by extension of a sinusitis or an otitis media.)
Secondary to Otitis Media, Mastoiditis, Lung Abscess	Penicillin G 10 million units/day IV plus third generation cephalosporin IV plus metronidazole
Post-traumatic	Cloxacillin or nafcillin plus third generation cephalosporin

In addition to beginning antibiotic medication, a patient with a subdural empyema or a brain abscess should be referred for neurosurgical assessment.

Prophylactic antiepileptic therapy should be administered routinely as follows: *phenytoin* (Dilantin) loading dose 18 mg/kg at a rate no faster than 25 to 50 mg/min followed by a maintenance dosage of 100 mg IV q8h or 300 mg PO daily. Steroid treatment for increased intracranial pressure due to cerebral edema should also be given routinely; *dexamethasone* (Decadron) 10 mg IV initially, followed by a maintenance dosage of 4 mg PO or IV q6h.

Selective History and Chart Review

Was the onset of the headache sudden or insidious?

The abrupt onset of a severe headache suggests a vascular cause, the most serious being subarachnoid hemorrhage.

How severe is the headache?

Most "tension headaches" are mild and not incapacitating. However, when migraine headaches are associated with severe pain, the patient may look sick.

Were there any prodromal symptoms?

Nausea and vomiting are associated with increased intracranial pressure but may also occur with migraine or angle-closure glaucoma. *Photophobia and neck stiffness* are associated with meningitis. The classic *visual aura* (scintillations, migratory scotomata, and blurred vision) that precedes a migraine headache is helpful in making the diagnosis, but the absence of these symptoms does not rule out migraine headache.

Is there a past history of chronic, recurring headaches?

Migraine and "tension" headaches follow a pattern. Ask the patient whether this headache is the same as their "usual headache"—the patient will probably make the diagnosis for you!

Is there a history of recent head trauma or alcohol abuse?

Subdural hematomas can appear insidiously 6 to 8 weeks after a seemingly minor trauma. There is an increased incidence of these in the alcoholic patient.

Has an ophthalmologist or another MD dilated the patient's pupils within the past 24 hours?

Acute angle–closure glaucoma can be precipitated by pupillary dilatation. The patient complains of a severe unilateral headache located over the brow and may experience nausea, vomiting, and abdominal pain.

Is there any decrease or loss in vision? Is there a history of jaw claudication?

Temporal arteritis is a systemic illness (low grade fever, malaise, weight loss, anorexia, weakness) seen in patients over 50 years of age. If this condition is suspected, order a stat ESR. Visual loss in temporal arteritis is a medical emergency and should be managed in consultation with a neurologist or rheumatologist. (For treatment see page 92).

What drugs is the patient receiving?

Drugs such as nitrates, calcium entry blockers, and indomethacin can cause headaches.

Selective Physical Examination II

VITALS   Repeat now.

HEENT   Red eye (acute angle–closure glaucoma)
        Hemotympanum or blood in the ear canal (basal skull fracture)
        Tender, enlarged temporal arteries (temporal arteritis)
        Retinal hemorrhages (hypertension)
        Lid ptosis, dilated pupil, eye deviated down and out (posterior communicating cerebral artery aneurysm)
        Tenderness on palpation or failure of transillumination of the frontal and maxillary sinuses (sinusitis or subdural empyema)
        Cranial bruit (arteriovenous malformation)
NEURO   Complete neurologic examination
        What is the level of consciousness?
        Drowsiness, yawning, or inattentiveness associated with headache are all ominous signs. In a patient with a small subarachnoid hemorrhage, these may be the only signs.
        Is there any *asymmetry* of pupils, visual fields, eye movements, limbs, tone, reflexes, or plantar responses? Asymmetry suggests structural brain disease. If this is a new finding, a CT scan of the head will be required.
MSS   Palpate skull and face looking for fractures, hematomas, and lacerations.
        Evidence of recent head trauma suggests the possibility of a subdural or an epidural hematoma.

Management II

Chronic Psychogenic Headaches. *Chronic psychogenic headaches* ("tension headaches," depression, anxiety) may be temporarily treated with non-narcotic analgesics. These are the commonest type of headaches you will see in the hospital. A long-term treatment plan, if not already established, may be discussed in the morning.

Mild Migraine Headaches. *Mild migraine headaches* can be treated adequately with aspirin or acetaminophen.

Severe Migraine Headaches. *Severe migraine headaches* are best treated immediately during the prodromal stage, but it is unlikely you will be called until the headache is well established. Ask the patient what they usually take for their migraine headache—it will probably be the most effective agent you can prescribe immediately. A severe migraine may require a narcotic analgesic agent, such as *codeine* 30 to 60 mg PO or IM q3 to 4h PRN or *meperidine* (Demerol) 50 to 100 mg IM q3 to 4h PRN.

If the patient usually takes ergotamine for migraine headaches, remember ergotamine is *contraindicated,* owing to its vasospastic effects, in the following situations:

- Peripheral vascular or coronary artery disease
- Hepatic or renal disease
- Hypertension
- Pregnancy

Cluster Headaches. *Cluster headaches* are difficult to treat. O_2 given at a flow rate of 7 L/min for 10 minutes may abort some cluster headaches. If this fails, *ergotamine* 2 mg PO or SL, initially, followed by 1 to 2 mg PO or SL q30 min until the attack has abated to a maximum of 6 mg/day (see previous discussion for contraindications) or narcotic analgesics (*codeine* 30 to 60 mg PO or IM q3 to 4h) may be tried.

Post-concussion Headaches. *Post-concussion headaches* (provided subdural and epidural hemorrhages have been ruled out by physical examination or by a CT scan of the head) should be treated with an analgesic agent which is unlikely to cause sedation, e.g., acetaminophen and codeine. Aspirin is contraindicated in the post-trauma patient; the inhibition of platelet aggregation may predispose the patient to bleeding complications.

Hemorrhages and Lesions. *Patients with subdural, epidural, and subarachnoid hemorrhages and space-occupying lesions* (brain abscess, tumor) causing raised intracranial pressure should be referred to a neurosurgeon as soon as possible.

Malignant Hypertension. *Malignant hypertension* (hypertension and papilledema) should be managed by careful reduction of BP (see Chapter 13, page 118).

Benign Intracranial Hypertension. *Benign intracranial hypertension* (pseudotumor cerebri) is a syndrome of unknown etiology with increased intracranial pressure (headache and papilledema) and no evidence of a mass lesion or hydrocephalus. Refer the patient to a neurologist in the morning for further investigation and management.

Temporal Arteritis. *Temporal arteritis* should be treated immediately to prevent irreversible blindness. *Prednisone* 60 mg PO daily can be started immediately when this diagnosis is suspected and supported by an ESR of > 60 mm/hr (Westergren's method). Confirmation by temporal artery biopsy should be arranged within the next 3 days.

Glaucoma. *A patient with acute angle–closure glaucoma* should be referred to an ophthalmologist immediately.

12

HEART RATE AND RHYTHM DISORDERS

There are only three abnormalities in heart rate or rhythm that you will be called to assess at night—*too fast, too slow, and irregular.* Remember that the main purpose of one's heart rate is to keep blood pressure high enough to perfuse the following three vital organs: (1) the heart, (2) the brain, and (3) the kidney. Your task is to find out why the heart is beating too quickly, too slowly, or irregularly before it results in hypoperfusion of the patient's vital organs. Begin by asking whether the heart rate is too fast or too slow. (Rapid heart rates are discussed subsequently; slow heart rates are addressed on page 107 of this chapter.) Next decide whether the rhythm is regular or irregular.

RAPID HEART RATES

Phone Call

Questions

1. **What is the heart rate?**
2. **Is the rhythm regular or irregular?**
3. **Is this a "new" problem since admission?**
4. **What is the BP?**
   Remember that hypotension may be a *cause* of tachycardia (i.e., compensatory), or a *result* of tachycardia that does not allow adequate diastolic filling of the left ventricle to maintain BP.
5. **Is the patient having chest pain or SOB?**
   Dysrhythmias are common in patients with underlying coronary artery disease. A rapid heart rate may be the result of angina or CHF or may precipitate angina or CHF in such a patient.
6. **What is the respiratory rate?**
   Any illness causing hypoxia may result in tachycardia.
7. **What is the temperature?**
   Tachycardia, proportionate to the temperature elevation, is an expected finding in a febrile patient. However, you must still examine the patient to make sure there is no other cause for the rapid heart rate.

Orders

1. If the patient is experiencing tachycardia and *hypotension,* order a large bore (size 16 if possible) IV immediately.

2. If the patient is having *chest pain,* ask the RN to put the cardiac arrest cart in the room and attach the patient to the ECG monitor.
3. Order a stat 12-lead ECG and rhythm strip.

Inform RN

"Will arrive at bedside in . . . minutes."

A rapid heart rate in association with chest pain (angina), shortness of breath (CHF), or hypotension requires you to see the patient immediately.

ELEVATOR THOUGHTS (What causes rapid heart rates?)

Rapid Irregular Heart Rates	Atrial fibrillation
	Multifocal atrial tachycardia
	Sinus tachycardia with PACs
	Sinus tachycardia with PVCs
Rapid Regular Heart Rates	Sinus tachycardia
	"Supraventricular tachycardia"
	—atrial flutter
	—paroxysmal atrial tachycardia
	Junctional tachycardia
	Ventricular tachycardia

Major Threat to Life

- *Hypotension,* leading to shock
- *Angina,* progressing to myocardial infarction
- *CHF,* leading to hypoxia

It is useful to recall the determinants of BP as expressed in the following two formulas:

Blood Pressure (BP) =
     Cardiac Output (CO) × Total Peripheral Resistance (TPR)

Cardiac Output (CO) = Heart Rate (HR) × Stroke Volume (SV)

As evidenced by the first formula, any fall in CO will result in a fall in BP. Although in most instances a rapid heart rate serves to increase CO, many of the "rapid heart rates" do not allow adequate time for diastolic filling of the ventricles, resulting in a low SV and, hence, a decreased CO. The low CO may result in *hypotension* (as may be seen in the formulas), in *angina* in the patient with underlying coronary artery disease, or in CHF in the patient with inadequate left ventricular reserve.

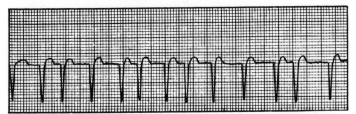

Figure 12–1. Atrial fibrillation with uncontrolled ventricular response.

Bedside

Quick Look Test

Does the patient look well (comfortable), sick (uncomfortable or distressed), or critical (about to die)?

Patients with tachycardia severe enough to cause hypotension usually look sick or critical. However, a patient with supraventricular or ventricular tachycardia may look deceptively well, if adequate BP is maintained.

Airway and Vital Signs

What is the heart rate? Is it regular or irregular?

Read the ECG and rhythm strip.

What is the blood pressure?

If hypotensive (systolic BP < 90 mm Hg), you must decide the following quickly:

- Whether the tachycardia is a result of the hypotension (i.e., a compensatory tachycardia).

OR

- The hypotension is a result of the tachycardia (i.e., inadequate diastolic filling leading to low CO with low BP). Three rapid heart rates can occasionally cause hypotension due to decreased diastolic filling, resulting in hypoperfusion of vital organs. These rhythms are atrial fibrillation with uncontrolled ventricular response, supraventricular tachycardia, and ventricular tachycardia (Fig. 12–1 to Fig. 12–3). If the patient is hypotensive, it is important to recognize these three rhythms immediately because prompt treatment is required to return the blood pressure to normal.

Management I

If the patient is *hypotensive* and has atrial fibrillation with uncontrolled ventricular response, supraventricular tachycardia, or ventricular tachycardia, emergency cardioversion may be required.

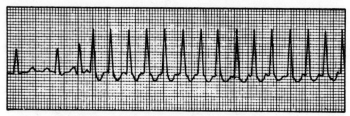

Figure 12–2. Supraventricular tachycardia.

- Ask the RN to call for your resident immediately.
- Ask the RN to bring the cardiac arrest cart into the room. Attach the patient to the ECG monitor.
- Ask the RN to draw *diazepam* (Valium) 10 mg IV into a syringe.
- Ensure that an IV is in place.

If the patient is *hypotensive* and none of these three rhythms is present, the tachycardia is most likely secondary to hypotension. You must perform a selective physical examination to decide which of the four major causes of hypotension is resulting in compensatory tachycardia: (1) cardiogenic causes, (2) hypovolemic causes, (3) sepsis, and (4) anaphylaxis. (Refer to Chapter 15 for investigation and management of hypotension.)

Fortunately, most of the patients you will see with rapid heart rates will not be hypotensive. In these cases, you may relax for a minute. Look at the ECG and rhythm strip and decide which rapid rhythm the patient is experiencing.

Rapid Irregular Rhythms

- Atrial fibrillation (Fig. 12–4)
- Multifocal atrial tachycardia (Fig. 12–5)
- Sinus tachycardia with PACs (Fig. 12–6)
- Sinus tachycardia with PVCs (Fig. 12–7)

Rapid Regular Rhythms

- Sinus tachycardia (Fig. 12–8)
- SVT: atrial flutter (Fig. 12–9)

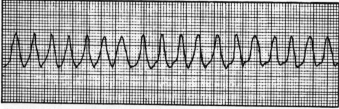

Figure 12–3. Ventricular tachycardia.

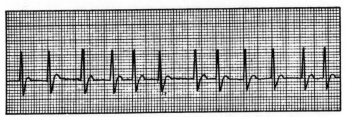

Figure 12–4. Rapid irregular rhythms. Atrial fibrillation.

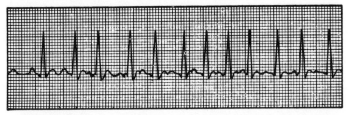

Figure 12–5. Rapid irregular rhythms. Multifocal atrial tachycardia.

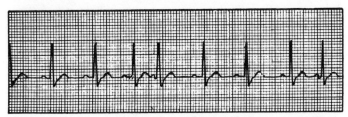

Figure 12–6. Rapid irregular rhythms. Sinus tachycardia with PACs.

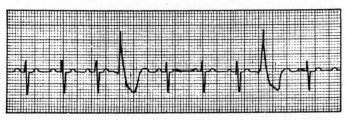

Figure 12–7. Rapid irregular rhythms. Sinus tachycardia with PVCs.

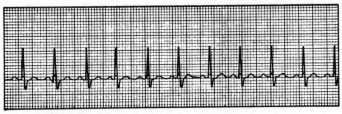

Figure 12–8. Rapid regular rhythms. Sinus tachycardia.

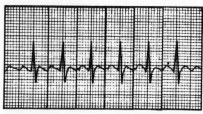

Figure 12–9. Rapid regular rhythms. SVT. Atrial flutter.

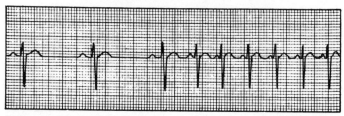

Figure 12–10. Rapid regular rhythms. SVT. Paroxysmal atrial tachycardia.

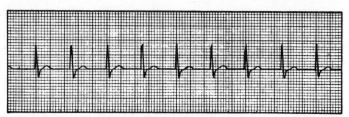

Figure 12–11. Rapid regular rhythms. SVT. Junctional tachycardia.

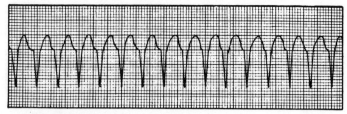

Figure 12–12. Rapid regular rhythms. Ventricular tachycardia.

- SVT: paroxysmal atrial tachycardia (Fig. 12–10)
- Junctional tachycardia (Fig. 12–11)
- Ventricular tachycardia (Fig. 12–12)

Management of Rapid Irregular Rhythms

Management of Atrial Fibrillation
If *unstable*—hypotensive, chest pain (angina) or SOB (CHF), and if atrial fibrillation is of recent onset (less than 3 days), the treatment of choice is cardioversion with 100 J.

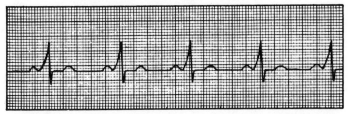

Figure 12–13. Wolff-Parkinson-White syndrome. This condition is characterized by a regular rhythm, a PR interval < 0.12 sec, a QRS complex > 0.11 sec, and a delta wave (i.e., slurred beginning of the QRS).

Atrial fibrillation with ventricular rates greater than 100/min and without evidence of hemodynamic compromise (no hypotension, angina, or CHF) can be treated with oral digoxin tablets. If the patient is not already receiving digoxin, give *digoxin* 0.25 mg PO q4h × 4 doses. Then, give 0.125 to 0.25 mg PO daily thereafter in a patient with normal renal function. In a patient already receiving digoxin, additional doses should be given with caution and careful observation.

Digoxin overdose is a common cause of morbidity in both community settings and hospital settings. Common side effects include dysrhythmias, heart blocks, GI upsets, and neuropsychiatric symptoms, such as hallucinations. It is unusual for these side effects to develop acutely, when digoxin is prescribed in the regimen previously outlined. The development of these side effects in the future can be minimized by adjusting maintenance digoxin doses according to renal function and by avoiding hypokalemia, which can predispose to digoxin toxicity.

Atrial fibrillation with ventricular rates less than 100/min in the untreated patient suggests underlying AV nodal dysfunction. These patients do not require treatment unless hemodynamically compromised (e.g., hypotension, angina, and CHF).

Once the ventricular rate is controlled, perform a *selective history and chart review* looking for the following causes of atrial fibrillation:

- Coronary artery disease
- Hypertension
- Hyperthyroidism (Check T_4.)
- Pulmonary embolism (Check for risk factors, see page 208.)
- Mitral or tricuspid valve disease (stenosis or regurgitation)
- Cardiomyopathy
- Congenital heart disease (e.g., atrial septal defect)
- Pericarditis
- Recent alcohol ingestion ("Holiday heart syndrome")
- Wolff-Parkinson-White syndrome (Fig. 12–13)
- Sick sinus syndrome

- Hypoxia
- Idiopathic ("lone fibrillator")

Selective Physical Examination

Look for specific causes of atrial fibrillation. Note that this process takes place *after* you have already begun to treat the patient.

VITALS   Repeat now.
HEENT   Exophthalmos, lid lag, lid retraction (hyperthyroidism)
RESP   Tachypnea, cyanosis, wheezing, pleural effusion (pulmonary embolus)
CVS   Murmur of mitral regurgitation or mitral stenosis (mitral valve disease)
EXT   Swelling, erythema, calf tenderness (DVT)

Management of Multifocal Atrial Tachycardia

This rhythm does not require specific management. One should treat the underlying cause, which is usually pulmonary disease and usually already being treated.

Check for the following underlying causes:

- Pulmonary disease (especially COPD)
- Hypoxia, hypercapnea
- Hypokalemia
- CHF
- Drugs
    Theophylline toxicity
    Digoxin toxicity
- Caffeine, tobacco, alcohol use

Multifocal atrial tachycardia can be a forerunner of atrial fibrillation.

Management of Sinus Tachycardia with PACs

Treatment is the same as that for multifocal atrial tachycardia. Again, PACs may be forerunners of multifocal atrial tachycardia or of atrial fibrillation, but PACs do not need to be treated unless atrial fibrillation develops.

Management of Sinus Tachycardia with PVCs

Look carefully at the ECG and rhythm strip and decide whether the PVCs are "malignant" or not as follows: *"R on T" phenomenon* (Fig. 12–14); *multifocal PVCs* (Fig. 12–15); *couplets or salvos* (three or more PVCs in a row) (Fig. 12–16); and *more than 5 PVCs/min* (Fig. 12–17).

Unless you can be certain that (1) the patient has not had an MI, (2) the patient is hemodynamically stable, and (3) the patient has had PVCs chronically, then the patient with "malignant" PVCs

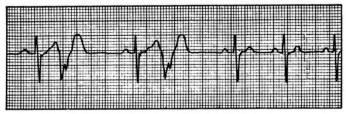

Figure 12–14. PVCs. "R on T" phenomenon.

should be transferred to the ICU/CCU for further investigation and continuous ECG monitoring.

Look for the following common causes of PVCs in the hospital:

- *Myocardial ischemia* (symptoms or signs of angina or MI). This is the most important cause of PVCs to identify, if present. PVCs are not generally associated with an increased risk of death unless they occur in the setting of myocardial ischemia.

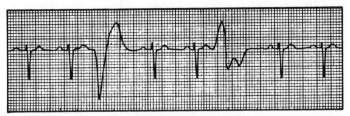

Figure 12–15. PVCs. Multifocal.

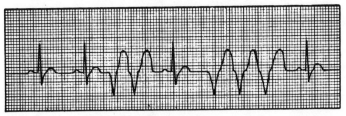

Figure 12–16. PVCs. Couplets or salvos.

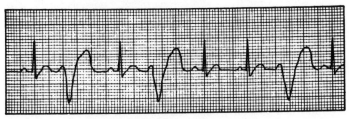

Figure 12–17. PVCs. More than 5/min.

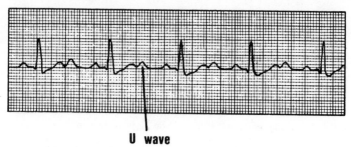

U wave

Figure 12–18. Electrocardiographic features of hypokalemia.

- *Hypokalemia.* Look for a recent serum potassium value in the chart, and order a repeat measurement if a recent one is not available. Check the 12-lead ECG for evidence of hypokalemia (Fig. 12–18). Ascertain whether the patient is on diuretics that may cause hypokalemia. (Refer to Chapter 27 for treatment.)
- *Hypoxia.* Obtain ABGs, if hypoxia is suspected clinically.
- *Acid base imbalance.* Obtain ABGs, if acidosis or alkalosis is suspected.
- *Cardiomyopathy.* Patients with cardiomyopathy severe enough to cause PVCs almost always have a cardiologist and an established diagnosis of cardiomyopathy before you see them. Therefore, consult the patient's cardiologist for guidance in treating cardiomyopathy-related PVCs.
- *Mitral valve prolapse.* Mitral valve prolapse can cause PVCs. Listen carefully for a systolic click and murmur. If "malignant" PVCs are not present, diagnosis can await confirmation by echocardiography in the morning.
- *Drugs.* Drugs, such as digoxin and other anti-arrhythmics, may actually *cause* PVCs.
- *Hyperthyroidism.* Look for signs of hypermetabolism, such as diaphoresis, tremor, heat intolerance, diarrhea, and ocular manifestations of hyperthyroidism, including lid lag, lid retraction, and exophthalmos. Order a serum T_4, if hyperthyroidism is suspected.

Try to identify whether any of the preceding eight factors are responsible for the PVCs and correct them, if possible.

Hypokalemia, hypoxia, and acid-base disturbances usually can be identified and corrected in the patient's room. However, if malignant PVCs are present or if there is suspicion of myocardial ischemia, cardiomyopathy, digoxin toxicity, or hyperthyroidism, the patient should be transferred to the ICU/CCU for continuous electrocardiographic monitoring and initiation of antiarrhythmics if indicated.

After the PVCs have been treated, the patient may still be left with *sinus tachycardia.* Investigation and management of the underlying sinus tachycardia should be undertaken as subsequently outlined.

Management of Rapid Regular Rhythms

Management of Sinus Tachycardia
There is no specific drug for the treatment of sinus tachycardia. The key is to find the *underlying cause* for this dysrhythmia. The most common causes in hospitalized patients of persistent sinus tachycardia are as follows:

- *Hypovolemia*
- *Hypotension* (cardiogenic, hypovolemic, sepsis, anaphylaxis). (Refer to Chapter 15 for investigation and management of hypotension.)
- *Shortness of breath* of any cause (CHF, pulmonary embolism, pneumonia, bronchospasm of COPD and asthma). (Refer to Chapter 20 for investigation and management of SOB.)
- *Fever*
- *Anxiety or pain*
- *Hyperthyroidism*
- *Drugs*

The treatment for sinus tachycardia is *always* treatment of the underlying cause.

Management of Supraventricular Tachycardias: Atrial Flutter
The treatment of atrial flutter is similar to that of atrial fibrillation. If *unstable,* the patient requires cardioversion; if *stable,* the patient may be treated with verapamil or digoxin IV (see page 105). Often, atrial flutter requires higher doses of digoxin than atrial fibrillation in order to slow the ventricular rate. Ironically, treatment of atrial flutter often produces atrial fibrillation.

Look for causes in the chart that may predispose the patient to atrial flutter. For the most part, these are the same diseases that can cause atrial fibrillation (see page 99).

Management of Supraventricular Tachycardia: Paroxysmal Atrial Tachycardia (PAT)
You will undoubtedly be anxious if called to see a patient with PAT who is unstable, because you know that may mean *cardioversion,* a technique with which you may not be familiar. Stay calm, there is still much you can do. If the patient is *unstable,* i.e., hypotensive, chest pain (angina), or SOB (CHF), prepare for immediate cardioversion as follows:

- Ask the RN to call for your resident immediately.
- Ask the RN to bring the cardiac arrest cart into the room. Attach the patient to the ECG monitor. Set the defibrillator to 25 J.

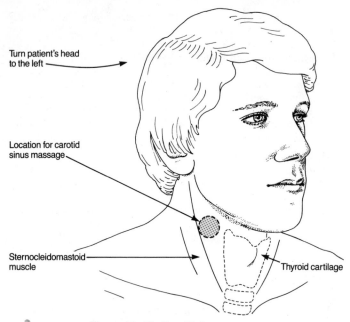

Figure 12–19. Carotid sinus massage.

- Ask the RN to draw *diazepam* (Valium) 10 mg IV into a syringe.
- Double check that an IV is in place.
- While waiting for the resident to arrive, try non-electrical means to convert the rhythm, e.g., Valsalva's maneuver, carotid sinus massage (see following section).

If the patient is hemodynamically stable, you may try one or more of the following:

- *Valsalva's maneuver.* Ask the patient to hold his or her breath and to "bear down as if you are going to have a bowel movement." This maneuver increases vagal tone and may terminate the PAT.
- *Carotid sinus massage.* This maneuver is an effective form of vagal stimulation and may thereby terminate PAT. It should always be performed with IV atropine available and with continuous ECG monitoring both for safety (some patients have developed asystole) and for documentation of results.

Listen over the carotid arteries for bruits and, if present, do not perform carotid sinus massage. If no bruit is heard, proceed as follows: Turn the patient's head to the left. Locate the carotid sinus just anterior to the sternocleidomastoid muscle at the level of the top of the thyroid cartilage (Fig. 12–19). Feel the carotid pulsation at this point and apply steady pressure to the carotid artery with two fingers for 10 to 15 seconds. Try the right side first and, if not effective, try the left side. Simultaneous bilateral massage of the carotid sinus should never be done, as you will effectively cut off cerebral blood flow!

Carotid sinus massage has resulted, on several occasions, in cerebral embolization of an atherosclerotic plaque from carotid artery compression. Although this is a rare complication, it can be minimized by first listening over the carotid artery for a bruit; if a bruit is heard one should forego carotid body massage on that side.

- Verapamil. If the dose, 2.5 to 5.0 mg IV over 5 minutes, is tolerated it can be repeated in 15 to 30 minutes when the response is not adequate. Verapamil increases AV conduction time and may slow ventricular rate.

Verapamil may cause hypotension if injected too rapidly. It is essential to give the dose slowly over 5 minutes. Verapamil is also a negative inotropic agent and may precipitate pulmonary edema in the patient with a predisposition to CHF.

- Digoxin. Provided the PAT is not due to digoxin toxicity (i.e., PAT with block), you may use *digoxin* 0.25 to 0.5 mg IV followed by 0.125 to 0.25 mg q4—6h until a full loading dose of 1 mg is given instead of verapamil. Then, a daily maintenance dose of 0.125 to 0.25 mg PO daily may be given if the patient has normal renal function.

Digoxin slows AV nodal conduction and may terminate PAT. The common side effects of digoxin (dysrhythmias, heart blocks, GI upsets, neuropsychiatric symptoms) are seldom acute when digoxin is prescribed in the regimen as outlined.

If the patient is known to have Wolff-Parkinson-White syndrome and is having rapid SVT, then *procainamide* is the drug of choice.

If hemodynamically stable and the aforementioned measures have not worked, the patient should be transferred immediately to the ICU/CCU for semi-elective cardioversion.

The underlying causes of supraventricular tachycardia are, for the most part, the same as those of atrial fibrillation and flutter (see page 99).

Management of Junctional Tachycardia

Occasionally a narrow, complex, regular tachycardia without P waves will be seen. This tachycardia is frequently associated with digoxin toxicity. Rapid rates from 120 to 180/min, if not associated with digoxin toxicity, can be treated the same as those for PAT (see above), through non-pharmacologic maneuvers, such as Valsalva's or carotid body massage, are much less likely to work.

Management of Ventricular Tachycardia

If the patient has no BP or pulse, call for a cardiac arrest and proceed with resuscitation as described on page 291.

If the patient is *unstable* (hypotensive, angina, or CHF) do the following:

- Call for the cardiac arrest cart and your resident immediately.
- Attach the patient to the ECG monitor.
- Make sure that an IV is in place.
- Order *lidocaine* 1 mg/kg IV to be given by syringe as rapidly as possible. At the same time begin a maintenance infusion of lidocaine at a rate of 1 to 4 to mg/min. In elderly patients and in patients with liver disease, CHF, or hypotension, give half the maintenance dose. In 5 to 15 minutes after the initial loading dose give a second bolus of lidocaine, 0.5 to 1 mg/kg IV. Lidocaine may cause drowsiness, confusion, slurred speech, and seizures—especially in the elderly and in patients with heart failure or liver disease. Once your patient has been transferred to the ICU/CCU, the staff there will need to watch carefully for these signs of lidocaine toxicity.
- *Cardioversion* at 50 J. Ventricular tachycardia with hemodynamic compromise or without prompt response to lidocaine requires cardioversion. A patient with an episode of ventricular tachycardia should be transferred to the ICU/CCU for continuous ECG monitoring.

After immediate resuscitation look for the following precipitating or potentiating causes of ventricular tachycardia:

- Ischemic heart disease (myocardial infarction, vasospasm, angina)
- Hypoxia
- Electrolyte imbalance (hypokalemia, hypomagnesemia, hypocalcemia)
- Hypovolemia
- Valvular heart disease (MVP)
- Acidemia
- Cardiomyopathy, CHF
- Drugs (digoxin toxicity)
    Quinidine
    Procainamide
    Disopyramide
    Phenothiazine
    Tricyclic antidepressants
    Amiodarone

These drugs may prolong the QT interval to produce a characteristic type of ventricular tachycardia known as torsades de pointes, which resembles a corkscrew pattern in the ECG rhythm strip, with complexes rotating above and below the baseline (Fig. 12–20). The drugs listed should be discontinued if such a rhythm develops, and lidocaine should be started as previously outlined.

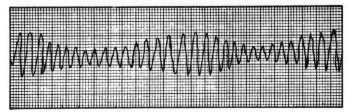

Figure 12–20. Torsades de pointes.

SLOW HEART RATES

Phone Call

Questions

1. **What is the heart rate?**
2. **What is the blood pressure?**
3. **Is the patient on digoxin, a beta blocker, or a calcium entry blocker?**
   Each drug may prolong AV nodal conduction and result in bradycardia due to heart block.

Orders

1. If the patient is hypotensive (systolic BP < 90 mm Hg), order an IV to be started immediately and ask the RN to place the patient in Trendelenburg's position (foot of the bed up). IV access is essential to deliver medications to increase the heart rate. Placing the patient in Trendelenburg's position achieves an "auto-transfusion" of 200 to 300 ml of blood.
2. If the heart rate is less than 40/min ask the RN to have a premixed syringe of *atropine* 1 mg ready at the bedside.
3. Stat ECG and rhythm strip.
4. Ask the RN to bring the cardiac arrest cart into the room and to attach the patient to the ECG monitor.

Inform RN

"Will arrive at bedside in . . . minutes."

"Bradycardia + hypotension" or any heart rate less than 50/min requires you to see the patient immediately.

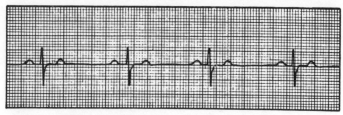

Figure 12–21. Slow heart rate. Sinus bradycardia.

ELEVATOR THOUGHTS (What causes slow heart rates?)

Sinus Bradycardia (Fig. 12–21)

DRUGS	Beta blockers
	Calcium entry blockers
	Digoxin
CARDIAC	Sick sinus syndrome
	Acute MI usually of inferior wall
	Vasovagal attack
MISC	Hypothyroidism
	Healthy young athletes
	Increased intracranial pressure in association with hypertension

Second Degree AV Block

Type I (Wenckebach's) (Fig. 12–22) and Type II (Fig. 12–23)

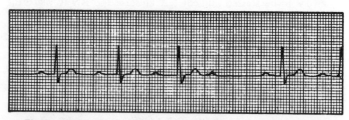

Figure 12–22. Slow heart rate. Second degree AV block (Type I).

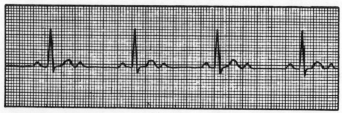

Figure 12–23. Slow heart rate. Second degree AV block (Type II).

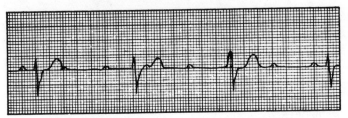

Figure 12–24. Slow heart rate. Third degree AV block.

DRUGS   Beta blockers
            Digoxin
            Calcium entry blockers
CARDIAC   Acute MI
            Sick sinus syndrome

Third Degree AV Block (Fig. 12–24)

DRUGS   Beta blockers
            Calcium entry blockers
            Digoxin
CARDIAC   Acute MI
            Sick sinus syndrome

Atrial Fibrillation with Slow Ventricular Rate (Fig. 12–25)

DRUGS   Digoxin
CARDIAC   Sick Sinus syndrome

Notice that no matter which bradycardia is present, the most common causes are drug-related and cardiac.

Major Threat to Life

- Hypotension
- Myocardial Infarction

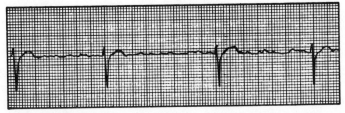

Figure 12–25. Atrial fibrillation with slow ventricular rate.

Two major threats to life exist in the patient with bradycardia as follows: first, if the heart rate is low enough it will result in hypotension due to inadequate CO, resulting in hypoperfusion of vital organs. A second concern is that if the bradycardia is due to MI, the patient will be prone to even more ominous dysrhythmias, such as ventricular tachycardia or fibrillation.

Bedside

Quick Look Test

Does the patient look well (comfortable), sick (uncomfortable or distressed), or critical (about to die)?

If the patient looks sick or terminal ask the RN to bring the cardiac arrest cart to the bedside and attach the patient to the ECG monitor. This may give instant diagnosis of the patient's rhythm, allow continuous monitoring, and provide instant feedback as to the effects of your intervention.

Airways and Vital Signs

What is the heart rate?

Read the ECG to identify which slow rhythm is occurring.

What is the blood pressure?

Most causes of hypotension are accompanied by a compensatory reflex *tachycardia*. If hypotension exists with any of the bradycardias, proceed as follows:

- Notify your resident as soon as possible.
- Elevate the legs. This is a temporary measure serving to empty the legs of blood volume and improve cardiac, cerebral, and renal perfusion.
- *Atropine* 0.5 mg IV as rapidly as possible.
- If no response after 5 minutes, given an additional 0.5 mg atropine IV q5 min up to a total dose of 2.0 mg IV.
- If still no improvement, begin an IV *isoproterenol* (Isuprel) infusion by adding 2 mg of isoproterenol to 500 ml D5W, running at 1 to 10 mcg/minute (15 to 150 ml/hr). Any patient receiving an isoproterenol infusion should be transferred to the ICU/CCU for further monitoring and possible pacemaker placement.

Selective History and Chart Review

Look for the cause of the bradycardia.

DRUGS   Beta blockers
               Calcium entry blockers
               Digoxin

CARDIAC ISCHEMIA	Does the patient have a history of angina or previous MI?
	Has there been any hint (chest pain, SOB, nausea, or vomiting) of a cardiac ischemic event occurring within the last few days?
	Does the patient have other evidence of atherosclerosis (previous stroke, TIAs, peripheral vascular disease) that may be a clue to the concomitant presence of coronary artery disease?
	Does the patient have current risk factors (hypertension, diabetes mellitus, smoking, hypercholesterolemia, family history of coronary artery disease) that may suggest that this is the first episode of cardiac ischemia?
	If there is any evidence of a possible acute myocardial infarction being responsible for the bradycardia, the patient should go to the ICU/CCU for ECG monitoring.
VASOVAGAL ATTACK	Is there a history of pain, straining, or other Valsalva-like maneuver immediately prior to occurrence of the bradycardia?
	This is only relevant in cases of sinus bradycardia. Heart blocks should never be attributed to a vasovagal attack.

Selective Physical Examination

Look for a cause of the bradycardia.

VITALS	Bradypnea (hypothyroidism)
	Hypothermia (hypothyroidism)
	Hypertension (risk factor for coronary artery disease)
HEENT	Coarse facial features (hypothyroidism)
	Loss of lateral third of eyebrows (hypothyroidism)
	Periorbital xanthomas (coronary artery disease)
	Fundi with hypertensive or diabetic changes (coronary artery disease)
	Carotid bruits (cerebrovascular disease with concomitant coronary artery disease)
CVS	New S_4 (nonspecific but common finding in acute MI)
ABD	Renal, aortic, or femoral bruits (concomitant coronary artery disease)
EXT	Poor peripheral pulses (peripheral vascular disease with concomitant coronary artery disease)
NEURO	Delayed return phase of deep tendon reflexes (hypothyroidism)

Management

Sinus Bradycardia

- No immediate treatment is required if the patient is not hypotensive.
- If on digoxin with an HR less than 60/min, further digoxin doses should be held until the HR is greater than 60/min.
- If the patient is on beta blockers and not hypotensive, no immediate treatment is required. However, with very slow heart rates (less than 40/min), one should hold the next dose of beta blocker until the HR is greater than 60/min and decrease the maintenance dose of beta blocker in consultation with the attending physician.

Second Degree AV Block (Type I and Type II) and Third Degree Block

Patients with either second or third degree heart blocks should be temporarily taken off any drugs which are known to prolong AV conduction, and transferred to a bed where continuous electrocardiographic monitoring is available.

Atrial Fibrillation with Slow Ventricular Response

This dysrhythmia does not require treatment unless the patient is hypotensive or has symptoms (syncope, confusion, angina, CHF) suggestive of vital organ hypoperfusion. Definitive treatment requires transfer to the ICU/CCU for pacemaker placement.

REMEMBER

1. Discontinuation of digoxin may mean that the original tachy-dysrhythmia or CHF for which the patient was being treated may return, if not closely monitored. Observe the patient closely over the next few days to ensure that tachydysrhythmia or CHF does not recur.
2. Abrupt discontinuation of beta blockers may result in rebound hypertension, angina, or MI. Again, observe the patient closely over the next several days. When the heart rate rises to > 60/min, the beta blocker may be reinstituted at a lower dosage. If treated in this manner, rebound hypertension or cardiac ischemia is seldom a problem.

13

HIGH BLOOD PRESSURE

Calls concerning high blood pressure are frequent at night. They rarely require the use of drugs that rapidly reduce the pressure. The level of the BP itself is of less importance than the rate of the rise and the setting in which the high BP is occurring.

PHONE CALL

Questions

1. **Why is the patient in the hospital?**
2. **Is the patient pregnant?**
   Hypertension in the pregnant patient may indicate the development of pre-eclampsia or eclampsia and should be assessed immediately.
3. **Is the patient taking antidepressant drugs?**
   Hypertension occurring in a patient receiving MAO inhibitors or tricyclics suggests a catecholamine crisis due to food or drug interaction.
4. **Is the patient in the emergency room?**
   Hypertension in young individuals presenting to the emergency room may becaused by catecholamine hypertension due to cocaine or amphetamine abuse.
5. **How high is the pressure and what has the pressure been previously?**
6. **Does the patient have symptoms suggestive of a "hypertensive emergency"?**

- Back and chest pain (aortic dissection)
- Chest pain (myocardial ischemia)
- Shortness of breath (pulmonary edema)
- Headache, neck stiffness (subarachnoid hemorrhage)
- Headache, vomiting confusion, seizures (hypertensive encephalopathy)
- Arterial bleeding from any site

7. **What anti-hypertensive medication is the patient taking now?**

ORDERS

If the patient has any symptoms of a "hypertensive emergency," order IV D5W TKVO immediately.

Inform RN

"Will be at bedside in . . . minutes."

Situations requiring immediate assessment and possibly prompt lowering of blood pressure include the following:

- Eclampsia
- Aortic dissection
- Pulmonary edema resistant to other emergency treatment (see Chapter 20, page 206)
- Coronary ischemia
- Catecholamine crisis
- Hypertensive encephalopathy

ELEVATOR THOUGHTS

The diagnosis of *pre-eclampsia* can be made in the obstetric patient with hypertension, edema, and proteinuria. This syndrome usually occurs in the third trimester of pregnancy, at which stage hypertension is defined as a BP of 140/85 mm Hg or greater for more than 4 to 6 hours or as an increase of 30 mm Hg in systolic or 15 mm Hg in diastolic pressure, or more, from the pregestational values.

Aortic dissection is potentiated by high shearing forces determined by the rate of rise of the intraventricular pressure as well as the systolic pressure.

Elevation of afterload (increased systemic vascular resistance and elevated blood pressure) may be a readily correctable detrimental factor in *coronary ischemia* and *pulmonary edema.*

Catecholamine crises can be caused by the following:

Drug overdoses	Cocaine and amphetamines
Drug interactions	MAO inhibitors and indirect acting catechols (wine, cheese, ephedrine)
	Tricyclics and direct acting catechols (epinephrine and norepinephrine)
Pheochromocytoma	

Hypertensive encephalopathy is a rare complication of hypertension and even more unusual in hospitalized patients. Vomiting developing over several days and headache, lethargy, or confusion are suggestive symptoms. Focal neurologic deficits are uncommon in the early course of encephalopathy.

BP fluctuates in normal individuals and more so in hypertensive individuals. Excitement, fear, and anxiety from unrelated medical conditions or procedures can cause marked transient increases in BP. BP measurements require care in regard to proper cuff size, proper cuff placement, and repeated measurements.

MAJOR THREAT TO LIFE

The major immediate threat to life is a marked increase in blood pressure with the following:

- Eclampsia
- Aortic dissection
- Pulmonary edema
- Myocardial infarction
- Hypertensive encephalopathy

BEDSIDE

Quick Look Test

Does the patient look well (comfortable), sick (uncomfortable or distressed), or critical (about to die)?

Unless the patient is having seizures (eclampsia, hypertensive encephalopathy) or is markedly SOB (pulmonary edema) the severity of the situation cannot be assessed by his or her initial appearance. The patient may be suffering from hypertensive encephalopathy yet look deceptively well.

Airway and Vital Signs

What is the BP?

Retake the blood pressure in both arms.

Accompanying arteriosclerosis may unilaterally reduce brachial artery flow and may give an artifactually low BP reading. A lower pressure in the left arm may be a clue to aortic dissection. Too small a cuff on an obese patient or a patient with rigid arteriosclerotic peripheral vessels may give readings that are factitiously high in relationship to the intra-arterial pressure.

What is the heart rate?

Bradycardia and hypertension in a patient not on beta blockers may indicate increasing intracranial pressure. Tachycardia and hypertension can be seen in "catecholamine crisis."

Selective History

Can the patient further elucidate the duration of hypertension? Ask the patient about any symptoms suggestive of a hypertensive emergency.

- Headache (an occipital headache or a neckache, lethargy, or visual blurring suggest, particularly, hypertensive encephalopathy)
- Chest pain (myocardial ischemia)

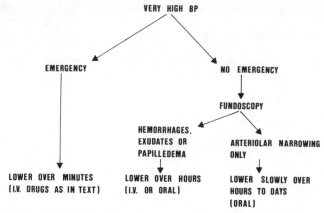

Figure 13–1. Approach to management of very high blood pressure.

- SOB (pulmonary edema)
- Back or chest pain (aortic dissection)

Unilateral weakness or sensory symptoms suggest a cerebrovascular accident. Such an episode in a previously hypertensive patient may be associated with a transient increase in BP.

Selective Physical Examination

Does the patient have evidence of a hypertensive emergency?

HEENT   Assess the fundi for hypertensive changes (generalized or focal arteriolar narrowing, flame-shaped hemorrhages near the disc, dot and blot hemorrhages, exudates)

Papilledema. If a hypertensive emergency (crisis) is not present, but fundi show hemorrhages, exudates, or papilledema, BP will still need to be lowered "urgently" over a period of *hours,* using either IV or oral medications. Patients with fundoscopic findings limited to arteriolar narrowing in the absence of a hypertensive emergency require even slower (over a matter of hours or days) BP control using oral treatment (Fig. 13–1).

RESP   Crackles, pleural effusion (CHF)
CVS   Elevated JVP, S_3 (CHF)
NEURO   Confusion, delirium
Agitation or lethargy (hypertensive encephalopathy)
Localized deficits (stroke)

Management

Most often the elevated BP will be an isolated finding in an asymptomatic patient known to have hypertension. Although long-

116

term control of hypertension in such patients is of proven benefit, acute lowering of pressure is not. Remember the risk of overshooting the mark in acute reduction of BP in patients with longstanding, high BP and high levels of autoregulation of cerebral blood flow. Do not treat a BP reading, treat the condition associated with it!

True emergencies require special management. These include the following:

- Hypertensive encephalopathy
- Malignant hypertension (marked elevation of diastolic pressure with fundal hemorrhages and exudates and usually some compromise in renal function)
- Eclampsia
- Subarachnoid or cerebral hemorrhage
- Aortic dissection
- Hypertension and pulmonary edema or myocardial ischemia
- Catecholamine crisis

Call your resident now for help if you are unfamiliar with the management of these conditions.

Hypertensive Encephalopathy. This is almost always accompanied by papilledema in addition to retinal exudates and hemorrhages. Focal neurologic deficits are unusual in the early part of the course and suggest a stroke. Remember, particularly, the risk of lowering pressure too quickly in patients with atherothrombotic cerebrovascular disease; you can precipitate a stroke!

1. Transfer the patient to the ICU/CCU for ECG monitoring and intra-arterial BP monitoring.
2. Notify the ICU/CCU staff that the patient will require an IV *nitroprusside infusion*. In most medical institutions, IV nitroprusside infusion cannot be given to patients in general medical units because of the requirement for intra-arterial blood pressure monitoring. However, you may expedite treatment by informing the ICU/CCU staff when patients will be requiring IV nitroprusside infusions.
3. Alternatively, *diazoxide* may be given in the patient's room under your resident's guidance in an emergency, such as hypertensive encephalopathy. Diazoxide is a direct arterial vasodilator and may be administered in the following regimen: *diazoxide* (Hyperstat) 50 mg IV injected over 3 min q15 min × two doses, while monitoring the BP q5 min. If ineffective, increase the dosage to 100 mg IV q15 min × two doses, until a total of 300 to 450 mg diazoxide has been given. A diazoxide infusion at a rate of 15 mg/min is another alternative that will usually effect a smooth reduction in blood pressure within 30 minutes. Because diazoxide causes reflex tachycardia and increases CO, it is contraindicated for the treatment of hypertension in the setting of acute MI, dissecting aortic aneurysm, or intracerebral hem-

orrhage. Because of its potent antidiuretic effect, it is also contraindicated in hypertension complicated by CHF. Diazoxide has also been observed to interrupt labor during treatment for pre-eclampsia. Side effects due to the too rapid lowering of the BP (reflex tachycardia, angina, cerebral ischemia) can be minimized by monitoring the BP closely and by discontinuing the IV bolus or infusion when the desired BP response is achieved.

4. *Labetalol* (Normodyne, Trandate) is a combined alpha and beta blocking agent that may be given intravenously without intra-arterial monitoring. It may be given in repeated incremental doses, beginning at 20 mg IV q10 to 15 min (e.g., 20 mg, 20 mg, 40 mg, 40 mg). Alternatively, a labetalol infusion beginning at 2 mg/min and titrating to a BP response may be given. Labetalol is not as useful in lowering BP if the patient is already on a beta blocker.

5. Since transfer to the ICU/CCU often takes longer than 30 minutes, you may temporarily achieve BP control by giving the patient *nifedipine* (Adalat) 5 to 10 mg PO × one dose. Patients with longstanding hypertension are at risk from abrupt reduction of BP, which may compromise coronary and cerebral blood flow. In the presence of atherosclerosis, this circumstance can result in MI or stroke. The risk can be reduced if nifedipine is given orally as the intact capsule in an initial dose of 5 to 10 mg. The effect of this dose is usually apparent in 30 minutes, and a repeat dose of 5 to 10 mg may be given if insufficient BP lowering has been achieved. Few situations require the more rapid but less predictable response that occurs after biting and swallowing the capsule or after its sublingual administration. Aim for diastolic BP levels of around 100 mm Hg.

6. Once BP control is achieved through parenteral means, the patient should be started on an appropriate oral regimen to maintain satisfactory BP control.

Malignant Hypertension. Unless accompanied by another feature (e.g., encephalopathy, pulmonary edema), you have more time to gain control of the BP. Control may be achieved by using a combination of orally effective antihypertensive drugs. Review the patient's current antihypertensive treatment. Increase to their maximum effective dose or add other agents. More aggressive approaches can wait until morning.

Pre-eclampsia and Eclampsia. Treatment in these patients is complicated by the risk from both the disorder and the treatment to the fetus and to the mother. The treatment of choice near term is *magnesium sulfate* until delivery of the baby can be effected. Treatment should be initiated only in consultation with the patient's obstetrician. Magnesium sulfate is given as an IV infusion: mix 16 gm of magnesium sulfate in 1 L of D5W and give a loading dose of 250 ml (4 gm) IV over 20 minutes. The maintenance dosage is 1 to 2 gm (62.5 to 125 ml) /hr or more, as required. Order a serum magnesium level every 4 hours, aiming for a serum magnesium level of 6 to 8 mmol/L. Local practice may well include other drug selections.

Subarachnoid or Cerebral Hemorrhage. Although there is no proof that lowering of pressure alters outcome, many neurologists will administer drugs to control elevated pressures in these situations. Unless you are familiar with the local practice, a neurologist should be consulted.

Aortic Dissection
1. Transfer the patient to the ICU/CCU for intra-arterial BP monitoring and control of blood pressure with parenteral drugs.
2. *Nitroprusside* is useful in the management of aortic dissection but should not be used without an accompanying beta blocker, which will reduce the rate of rise of intraventricular pressure and hence the shearing force. These beta blockers should be given parenterally and high doses may be required as follows: *Propranolol*—0.5 mg IV followed by 1 mg IV q5 min until the pulse pressure is reduced to 60 mm Hg or to a total dose of 0.15 mg/kg, in any 4-hour period, with a maintenance dosage of q4 to 6h, or *labetalol* alone may be used for aortic dissection in the same regimen as for hypertensive encephalopathy (see page 118).

Hypertension and Pulmonary Edema or Myocardial Ischemia
1. In addition to BP control, pulmonary edema should be treated with the measures outlined in Chapter 20, page 206.
2. Transfer the patient to the ICU/CCU for continuous ECG and intra-arterial BP monitoring.
3. Notify the ICU/CCU staff that the patient will require an IV *nitroglycerin infusion.* Experimental evidence suggests that IV nitroglycerin is preferable to IV nitroprusside for the control of BP in a patient with myocardial ischemia, as nitroprusside may cause a coronary steal phenomenon, resulting in extension of the ischemic zone. It is therefore preferable to attempt control of the BP in a cardiac patient with IV nitroglycerin and, if unsuccessful, IV nitroprusside.

"Catecholamine Crisis." Pheochromocytoma is the classic condition ("pallor, palpitations, and perspiration") associated with intermittent and alarmingly high blood pressures. Other conditions associated with similar, sudden, and severe increase in blood pressures include cocaine and amphetamine abuse, clonidine withdrawal, and food (cheese), drug (ephedrine), and drink (wine) interactions with MAO inhibitors (antidepressants). Currently used

MAO inhibitors include tranylcypromine sulfate (Parnate), phenelzine sulfate (Nardil), and isocarboxazid (Marplan). If sudden increases in pressure are observed in patients on these drugs, the most likely cause is an interaction with a substance that is releasing the stores of catecholamines, which are overabundant because of inhibition of one of the catecholamine metabolizing enzymes (MAO).

1. Transfer the patient to the ICU/CCU for ECG and intra-arterial BP monitoring.
2. Notify the ICU/CCU staff that the patient will require special parenteral antihypertensive drugs.
3. *Phentolamine mesylate* may be given intravenously for marked elevation of BP. This drug causes a decrease in peripheral resistance and an increase in venous capacity, owing to a direct action on vascular smooth muscle. This effect may be accompanied by cardiac stimulation with tachycardia that is more than can be explained as a reflex response to peripheral vasodilation. In an emergency 2.5 to 5 mg may be given intravenously. However, if time permits, and for continuous control, phentolamine mesylate should be given at an initial dosage of 5 to 10 mcg/kg/min by continuous IV infusion.
4. In cocaine-induced hypertension *propranolol* 1 to 3 mg q2 to 5 min intravenously to a maximum of 8 mg is useful in reversing hypertension and tachycardia.
5. In amphetamine-induced hypertension *chlorpromazine* 1 mg/kg intramuscularly can reverse hypertension and hyperactivity.

14

HYPNOTICS, LAXATIVES, ANALGESICS, AND ANTIPYRETICS

Phone calls regarding the reordering of hypnotic, laxative, analgesic, and antipyretic medications are frequent. The majority of these requests can be managed over the phone.

HYPNOTICS

Phone Call

Questions

1. **Why is a hypnotic being requested?**
   The majority of requests for nighttime sedation are because of insomnia. Sleeping pills should not be prescribed for restless or agitated patients who have not been examined.
2. **Has the patient received hypnotics before?**
3. **What are the vital signs?**
4. **What was the reason for admission?**
5. **Does the patient have any of the following conditions in which hypnotics are contraindicated?**

- Depression
  An antidepressant is the drug of choice if insomnia is a manifestation of depression.
- Confusion
- Hepatic or respiratory failure
- Sleep apnea
- Myasthenia gravis

6. **Is the patient receiving other centrally active drugs that may interact, e.g., alcohol, antidepressants, antihistamines, narcotics?**
7. **Does the patient have any drug allergies?**
   The major contraindication to a specific hypnotic is a known allergy to the drug.

Orders

A benzodiazepine is the drug of choice for short-term treatment of insomnia. Sedative effects are comparable among all benzodiazepines; only the onset and duration of the effects differ. Table 14–1 lists the drug doses of various benzodiazepines.

Table 14–1. HYPNOTICS

	Peak Time (hr)	Biologic Half-life (hr)	Dose (QHS)*
Sedatives with the Most Rapid Onset			
Diazepam (Valium)	1.5–2	50–100	5–10 mg PO
Flurazepam (Dalmane)	1.0	50–100	15–30 mg PO
Lorazepam (Ativan)	1.0–6	12–25	1–2 mg PO or SL
Sedatives with the Shortest Duration			
Triazolam (Halcion)	2	2–3	0.25–0.5 mg PO
Oxazepam (Serax)	1–4	4–13	15–30 mg PO
Lorazepam (Ativan)	1–6	12–15	1–2 mg PO or SL

*Dose in elderly patients should ordinarily be half the usual adult dose.

Inform RN

"Will arrive at the bedside in . . . minutes."

Agitated, restless patients should be assessed before hypnotics are prescribed.

Remember

1. The half-lives of benzodiazepines vary from 2 to 3 hours for triazolam (Halcion) to 50 to 100 hours for diazepam (Valium). Accumulation can occur if the second and subsequent doses of drugs are given before the previous dose has been metabolized and excreted. Diazepam (Valium) and flurazepam (Dalmane) have active metabolites; the half-lives stated in Table 14–1 include the active metabolites.

   When these drugs are prescribed once or twice, the half-life of the drug is of no great concern. However, repeated use of benzodiazepines must take into account the individual drug's half-life; flurazepam (Dalmane) given repeatedly will cause a daytime "hangover," whereas triazolam (Halcion) will not. However, the shorter acting drugs may be associated with early morning insomnia and rebound daytime anxiety.

2. Benzodiazepines should not be prescribed on a continuous nightly basis but should be discontinued temporarily once one or two nights of acceptable sleep have been achieved. Using benzodiazepines for less than 14 consecutive nights helps to prevent the development of drug tolerance and dependence.

3. Be aware of the adverse effects of any drug you prescribe. The *adverse effects of benzodiazepines* are CNS depression (tiredness, drowsiness, "detached feeling"); headache, dizziness, ataxia, confusion, disorientation in the elderly; and psychologic dependence.

4. Barbiturates and non-barbiturate hypnotics, other than benzodiazepines, usually carry more risks than advantages as hypnotics and should be avoided.

Table 14–2. LAXATIVES AND ENEMAS

Laxatives

Bulk Forming Laxatives
Example: *Psyllium* (Metamucil)
  Onset: 24 hours
  Caution: May lead to intestinal obstruction in immobilized patients.
  Usual adult dose: 3 to 6 gm 1 to 3 times daily PO
  Use: General purpose—effect similar to high fiber diet.
Stool Softener
Example: *Docusate* (Colace)
  Onset: 24 to 72 hours
  Caution: No value in atonic colon.
  Usual adult dose: 100 to 200 mg PO BID
  Use: Give orally to avoid straining at stool (postpartum, MI).
Lubricants
Example: *Mineral Oil*
  Onset: 48 to 72 hours
  Caution: Do not use in a patient in whom a decreased level of consciousness
      makes aspiration a risk. Reduces absorption of fat soluble vitamins
      (A, D, E, and K).
  Usual adult dose: Plain 15 to 45 ml 1 to 2 times a day PO.
              Emulsion, 15 ml twice daily.
  Use: Routine use not recommended.
Stimulant Laxatives
Example: *Bisacodyl* (Dulcolax)
  Onset: 6 to 10 hours PO
      15 to 60 minutes PR
  Caution: Avoid in pregnancy, MI. Commonly overused leading to "laxative abuse
      colon." May worsen orthostatic hypotension, weakness, and
      incoordination in the elderly.
  Usual adult dose: 5 to 10 mg PO
              10 mg by suppository PR
  Use: Occasional use in acute constipation due to opiates, with prolonged bed rest
      and preparation for surgical, radiologic, or colonoscopic procedures.
Example: *Glycerin* Suppository
  Onset: 2 to 60 minutes
  Caution: Not intended for regular use
  Usual adult dose: 2.7 gm (1 suppository) PR
  Use: Acute emptying of the bowel prior to diagnostic procedures; acute
      constipation.
Osmotic Laxatives
Example: *Magnesium Hydroxide* (Milk of Magnesia)
  Onset: 1 to 8 hours
  Caution: Up to 20% of magnesium may be absorbed. Do not use in renal failure.
  Usual adult dose: 30 to 60 ml (approximately 2 to 4 gm) PO suspension (7 to 8.5
              gm/100 ml).
  Use: Acute emptying of the bowel prior to diagnostic procedures; acute
      constipation.

Table continued on following page

LAXATIVES

Laxatives are overused by the public at large. However, hospitalized patients require laxatives in certain circumstances as follows: after acute MI to limit straining; during the administration of narcotics; during prolonged bed rest; and during the evacuation of the bowels prior to abdominal surgery and some GI diagnostic procedures. The solutions employed in *enemas* have either hyper-

Table 14–2. LAXATIVES AND ENEMAS *Continued*

Enemas

Example: *Sodium Phosphate and Sodium Biphosphate* (Fleet enema)
  Onset: Immediate
  Caution: Do not use when nausea, vomiting, or abdominal pain is present.
  Usual adult dose: 60 to 120 ml (6 gm sodium phosphate and 16 gm sodium
                    biphospate/100 ml). (Available in a disposable plastic
                    container.)
  Use: Acute evacuation of the bowel prior to diagnostic procedures; acute
       constipation.
Example: *Bisacodyl* (Fleet Bisacodyl)
  Onset: Immediate
  Caution: Do not use when nausea, vomiting, or abdominal pain is present. Avoid
           in pregnancy and MI. May worsen orthostatic hypotension, weakness,
           and incoordination in the elderly.
  Usual adult dose: 37.5 ml (10 mg/30 ml). (Available in disposable plastic
                    containers.)
  Use: Acute evacuation of the bowel prior to diagnostic procedures; acute
       constipation.
Example: *Mineral Oil* (Fleet Mineral Oil Enema)
  Onset: Immediate
  Caution: Do not use when nausea, vomiting, or abdominal pain is present.
  Usual adult dose: 60 to 120 ml. (Available in disposable plastic containers.)
  Use: Impacted feces.

tonic properties, to stimulate rectal peristalsis, or have surfactant properties to achieve softening of impacted feces.

Phone Call

Questions

1. **Why is a laxative being requested?**
   The frequency of bowel movements is highly variable in the normal population, ranging from twice daily to once every 3 days. Make certain you know what this patient's normal bowel pattern is before prescribing a laxative.
2. **Has the patient received laxatives before? If so, which ones have been tried so far?**
3. **What are the vital signs?**
4. **What was the reason for admission?**
5. **When was a rectal examination last performed?**
   Fecal impaction, which requires a rectal examination for diagnosis (and sometimes for treatment!) is a relative contraindication to oral laxative use.
6. **Does the patient have nausea, vomiting, or abdominal pain?**
   These symptoms suggest an acute GI disorder.

Orders

Table 14–2 lists the drug doses of selected laxatives and enemas. Bowel movements can be increased in frequency by liquefying the stool; both bulk and osmotic laxatives increase the water content in the intestine. An increase in the frequency of bowel movements can also be induced by stool softeners and colon-irritating drugs that increase peristalsis.

Inform RN

"Will arrive at the bedside in . . . minutes."

The only time you need to assess a patient when a laxative has been requested is when the patient has associated nausea, vomiting, or abdominal pain or when fecal impaction is suspected. (See Chapter 4 for the assessment and management of abdominal pain.)

Remember

1. When a patient is constipated (unless there is fecal impaction) an oral laxative is the treatment of choice. If the oral laxative fails, a stronger-acting laxative can be used, and, failing this, a suppository is prescribed next. Lastly, enemas can be used as follows: first, a hypertonic enema solution (e.g., Fleet) and last, an oil retention enema.
2. When there is fecal impaction, an oil-based enema is the treatment of choice.
3. Soapsuds enemas are no longer used; they have been replaced by hypertonic enema solutions.

ANALGESICS

Most hospital pharmacies do not allow narcotic medication orders to stand indefinitely. Narcotic medications need to be re-ordered every 3 to 5 days, depending on the individual medical institution. Consequently, if the house staff fail to re-order these medications during the day, you may be called to do so at night.

Phone Call

Questions

1. **Why is an analgesic being requested?**
   The majority of requests are for re-ordering of medications.
2. **How severe is the pain?**
   This question will help to determine whether a non-narcotic analgesic may be sufficient.
3. **Is this a new problem?**
   The new onset of undiagnosed pain requires you to assess the patient, at the bedside, before ordering an analgesic medication.
4. **What are the vital signs?**

Table 14–3. ANALGESICS

Non-Narcotic Analgesics

Acetaminophen
  Onset: 30 minutes
  Caution: Do not use when the patient has known allergy to acetaminophen, liver
      failure, or G-6-PD.
  Drug interactions: None reported.
  Usual adult dose: 325 to 650 mg q4 to 6h PO
              650 mg q4 to 6h PR
              15 to 30 ml (120 mg/5 ml) elixir q4 to 6h PO
  Use: Pain of mild to moderate severity
Aspirin
  Onset: 30 minutes
  Caution: Do not use when there is known allergy to aspirin or other NSAID,
      recent peptic ulcer disease, coagulation abnormalities, or nasal polyps
      and asthma syndrome.
  Drug Interactions: Anticoagulants (warfarin, heparin)
              Sulfinpyrazone (Anturan), methotrexate,
              Acetazolamide (Diamox), probenecid (Benemid),
              Sulfonylureas
  Usual adult dose: 325 to 650 PO mg q4h
  Use: Mild to moderate pain.

Narcotics Analgesics

Codeine Phosphate
  Onset: 20 to 30 minutes
  Caution: Do not use when there is known allergy, undiagnosed pain, "surgical
      abdomen," hepatic encephalopathy, acute colitis, respiratory failure,
      pregnancy, chronic pain not secondary to terminal disease, or
      documented narcotic abuse or dependency. Use with caution in the
      elderly; they are prone to constipation.
  Drug interactions: CNS depressants
  Usual adult dose: 30 to 60 mg q4 to 6h PO, SC, or IM.
  Use: Useful when an oral narcotic agent is required for severe pain. Head
      injuries (since it has less sedative properties than other narcotics).
Meperidine (Demerol)
  Onset: 20 minutes
  Caution: See codeine phosphate.
  Drug interactions: CNS depressants. Contraindicated in patients receiving MAO
              inhibitors, e.g., phenelzine (Nardil), tranylcypromine
              (Parnate), or isocarboxazid (Marplan).
  Usual adult dose: 50 to 100 mg IM or SC q3 to 4h (up to 150 mg for severe
              pain).
  Use: Severe pain and post-operative pain while the patient is NPO.
Morphine
  Onset: 20 minutes
  Caution: See codeine phosphate. Contraindicated in pancreatitis and cholecystitis.
  Drug interactions: CNS depressants
  Usual adult dose: 5 to 10 mg IM or SC q4h. (For severe pain, 12 to 15 mg IM or
              SC q4h.)
  Use: Severe pain and postoperative pain while the patient is NPO.

The onset of fever in association with pain suggests a localized infectious process.

5. **What was the reason for admission?**
6. **Does the patient have any drug allergies?**

Orders

See Table 14–3 for drug dosages of selected analgesics.

Inform RN

"Will arrive at bedside in . . . minutes."

Any undiagnosed pain, new onset of severe pain, or change in character of previous pain requires you to assess the patient at the bedside, prior to ordering an analgesic.

Remember

If reversal of a narcotic overdose is required, the following are recommended:

1. *Reversal of post-operative narcotic depression.* Naloxone (Narcan) 0.2 to 2.0 mg IV q5 min until the desired improved level of consciousness is achieved (maximum total dose 10 mg). Doses q1 to 2h may be required to maintain reversal of CNS depression.
2. *Reversal of suspected narcotic overdose.* If the patient is comatose, intubation for airway protection should be undertaken prior to reversal; abrupt reversal may induce nausea and vomiting with the attendant risk of aspiration pneumonia. Give *naloxone* (Narcan) 0.2 mg IV SC or IM q5 min for several doses. If the initial dosage is ineffective, the dose may be increased incrementally to a maximum total dose of 10 mg.

Adverse Effects of Abrupt Narcotic Reversal. Nausea and vomiting, if provoked in the patient with an unprotected airway, may result in aspiration pneumonia. Hypertension and tachycardia can occur during narcotic reversal and may result in CHF in the patient with poor left ventricular function.

ANTIPYRETICS

Antipyretics should not be prescribed in the adult patient with fever unless the cause of the fever is known or the patient is symptomatic from the fever itself. (Refer to Chapter 9 for the approach to the febrile patient. Table 14–3 lists the dosages and side effects of acetaminophen and aspirin.)

15

HYPOTENSION AND SHOCK

Hypotension is a common call at night. Don't panic. Remember that hypotension does not become shock until there is evidence of inadequate tissue perfusion. An adequate BP is required to perfuse three vital organs—the *brain, heart,* and *kidneys.* Some patients normally have systolic blood pressures in the range of 85 to 100 mm Hg. The BP is adequate as long as the patient is not confused, disoriented, or unconscious; is not having angina; and is passing urine. By the same token, however, a BP of 105/70 mm Hg may result in serious hypoperfusion in a patient who is normally hypertensive.

PHONE CALL

Questions

1. **What is the BP?**
2. **What is the HR?**
3. **What is the temperature?**
   "Fever + hypotension" suggests impending septic shock.
4. **Is the patient conscious?**
5. **Is the patient having chest pain?**
6. **Is there evidence of bleeding?**
7. **Has the patient been given IV contrast material or an antibiotic within the last 6 hours?**
   If you are called to see a hypotensive patient in the x-ray department or a patient who has recently returned to the room from an x-ray procedure involving the administration of IV contrast material, your primary thought should be that the patient may be having an anaphylactic reaction.
8. **What was the admitting diagnosis?**

Orders

1. If the information provided over the telephone supports the possibility of impending or established shock, order the following:
   a. A large bore (#16 if possible) IV immediately, if not already in place. IV access is a high priority in the hypotensive patient.
   b. Place the patient in reverse Trendelenburg's position (i.e., head of the bed down and foot of the bed up). Although

hypotension should be assessed immediately, if you are unable to get to the bedside for 10 to 15 minutes, also ask the nurse to give 500 ml NS IV as rapidly as possible.

c. ABG tray at bedside
   Identification and correction of hypoxia and acidemia are essential in the management of shock.

2. If there is suspicion of *anaphylaxis,* ask the RN to have a pre-mixed syringe of IV epinephrine from the cardiac arrest cart available.

3. If the admitting diagnosis is *GI bleed* or there is visible evidence of blood loss
   a. Ensure that the patient has blood "on hold." If not, order a stat cross-match for 2, 4, or 6 units of packed RBCs depending on your estimate of blood loss.
   b. Hb stat. *Caution*: The Hb may be normal during an acute hemorrhage and drop only with correction of the intravascular volume by a shift of fluid from the extracellular space or by fluid therapy. (Refer to Chapter 10 for further investigation and management of GI bleeds.)

4. If an arrhythmia or ischemic myocardial event is suspected, order a stat ECG and rhythm strip. These may help you identify a rapid heart rhythm or an acute MI, which may be responsible for hypotension.

Inform RN

"Will arrive at bedside in . . . minutes."
Hypotension requires you to see the patient immediately.

ELEVATOR THOUGHTS (What causes hypotension or shock?)

- Cardiogenic causes
- Hypovolemia
- Sepsis
- Anaphylaxis

Two formulas, as follows, are useful to remember when considering the causes of hypotension:

$$\begin{array}{ccccc} \text{Blood pressure} & = & \text{cardiac output} & \times & \text{total peripheral resistance} \\ \text{(BP)} & = & \text{(CO)} & \times & \text{(TPR)} \end{array}$$

$$\begin{array}{ccccc} \text{Cardiac output} & = & \text{heart rate} & \times & \text{stroke volume} \\ \text{(CO)} & = & \text{(HR)} & \times & \text{(SV)} \end{array}$$

From these formulas it can be seen that hypotension results from either a fall in cardiac output or total peripheral resistance. "Cardiogenic causes" result from a fall in cardiac output due to either a fall in heart rate (e.g., heart block) or a fall in stroke volume (e.g., pump failure). Hypovolemia reduces stroke volume and hence cardiac output falls. Sepsis and anaphylaxis cause hypotension by lowering TPR.

MAJOR THREAT TO LIFE

Shock

Remember that hypotension does not become shock until there is evidence of inadequate tissue perfusion. As you will see, shock is a relatively easy diagnosis to make. Your goal is to identify and correct the cause of hypotension before it results in hypoperfusion of vital organs.

BEDSIDE

Quick Look Test

Does the patient look well (comfortable), sick (uncomfortable or distressed), or critical (about to die)?
A patient with hypotension but adequate tissue perfusion usually looks well. However, once perfusion of vital organs becomes compromised, the patient will look sick or critical.

Airway and Vital Signs

Is the airway clear?
If the patient is obtunded and cannot protect his or her airway, endotracheal intubation will be required. Ask the RN to notify the ICU/CCU immediately. Roll the patient onto the left side to avoid aspiration until intubation is achieved.

Is the patient breathing?
Assess respiration by checking the respiratory rate, chest expansion, and auscultation. All patients in shock should receive high flow oxygen.

Assess the circulation.
1. Examine for postural changes. A postural rise in HR > 15 beats/min, a fall in systolic BP > 15 mm Hg, or any fall in diastolic BP indicates significant hypovolemia.
2. Time the HR. Most causes of hypotension are accompanied by a compensatory reflex sinus tachycardia. If the patient is experiencing bradycardia or if you suspect a rhythm other than sinus tachycardia, refer to page 110 for bradycardia and page 95 for rhythm for further evaluation and management.

3. **Is the patient in *shock?*** This should take less than 20 seconds to determine.

VITALS   Repeat now.
CVS   Pulse volume, JVP
         Skin temperature and color
         Capillary refill
NEURO   Mental status
         Shock is a clinical diagnosis: systolic BP < 90 mm Hg with evidence of inadequate tissue perfusion, e.g., of the skin (cold, clammy, and cyanotic) and of the CNS (agitation, confusion, lethargy, coma). In fact, the kidney is a sensitive indicator of shock (urine output < 20 ml/hr), but immediate placement of Foley's catheter should not take priority over resuscitation measures.

What is the temperature?

An elevated temperature *or* hypothermia (< 36°C) suggests sepsis. However, remember that sepsis may appear in some patients, especially the elderly, with a normal temperature; hence, the absence of fever does not rule out the possibility of septic shock.

Look at the ECG and take the pulse:

Bradycardia. If the resting HR is < *50/min* in the presence of hypotension, suspect one of three things as follows:
1. Vasovagal Attack. If this is the case, the patient is usually normotensive by the time you arrive. Look for retrospective evidence of straining, Valsalva's maneuver, pain, or some other stimulus to vagal outflow. If vasovagal attack is suspected and there is persistent bradycardia despite leg elevation, give *atropine* 0.5 mg IV. If not effective, the same dose may be repeated q5 min up to a total dose of 2 mg IV.
2. Autonomic Dysfunction. The patient may be on a beta blocker and has been given too much, resulting in hypotension, or is hypotensive for some other reason but is unable to generate a tachycardia because of beta blockade, underlying sick sinus syndrome, or autonomic neuropathy. If the systolic BP is < 90 mm Hg administer atropine 0.5 mg IV. If not effective, the same dose may be repeated q5 min up to a total dose of 2 mg IV.
3. Heart Block. The patient may be suffering from a heart block (e.g., acute MI). Obtain a stat ECG to document the dysrhythmia. If systolic BP is < 90 mm Hg administer *atropine* 0.5 mg IV. If not effective, the same dose may be repeated q5 min up to a total dose of 2 mg IV. Refer to Chapter 12 for further investigation and management of heart block.

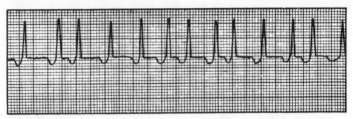

Figure 15–1. Atrial fibrillation with uncontrolled ventricular response.

Tachycardia. A compensatory sinus tachycardia is an expected, appropriate response in the hypotensive patient. Ensure by looking at the ECG that the patient does not have one of the following three rapid heart rhythms that may themselves cause hypotension due to decreased diastolic filling:

1. Atrial fibrillation with uncontrolled ventricular response (Fig. 15–1).
2. Supraventricular tachycardia (Fig. 15–2).
3. Ventricular tachycardia (Fig. 15–3).

If any one of these three rhythms is present in the hypotensive patient

- Ask the RN to notify your resident immediately.
- Ask the RN to bring the cardiac arrest cart into the room.
- Attach the patient to the ECG monitor.
- Ask the RN to draw up *diazepam* (Valium) 10 mg IV in a syringe.

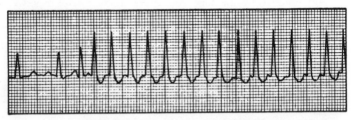

Figure 15–2. Supraventricular tachycardia.

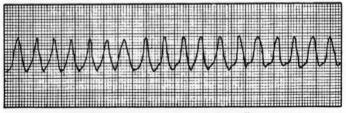

Figure 15–3. Ventricular tachycardia.

■ Ensure that an IV is in place. (Refer to Chapter 12, page 95, for further treatment of rapid heart rates associated with hypotension.)

Selective Physical Examination

Determine the *cause* of hypotension or shock by asking yourself two vital questions as follows:

What is the volume status?

Only cardiogenic shock will result in a clinical picture of *volume overload*. Hypovolemic, septic, or anaphylactic shock will all result in a clinical picture of *volume depletion*.

VITALS	Repeat now.
HEENT	Elevated JVP (CHF), flat neck veins (volume depletion)
	Angioedema (anaphylaxis)
RESP	Stridor (anaphylaxis)
	Crackles ± pleural effusions (CHF)
	Wheezes (anaphylaxis, CHF)
CVS	Cardiac apex displaced laterally, S_3 (CHF)
ABD	Hepatomegaly with positive HJR (CHF)
EXT	Presacral or ankle edema (CHF)
SKIN	Urticaria (anaphylaxis)
RECTAL	Melena or hematochezia (GI bleed)

Remember that *wheezing* may be seen in both CHF and anaphylaxis; administration of epinephrine may save the life of someone with anaphylaxis but may kill someone with CHF. Anaphylactic shock comes on relatively suddenly and nearly always an inciting factor (e.g., IV contrast material, penicillin) can be identified. Usually, other clues such as angioedema or urticaria are present.

Management

What immediate measures need to be taken to correct or prevent shock from occurring?

Normalize the intravascular volume. In the case of *cardiogenic shock* (volume overload), stop the IV NS bolus (ordered over the phone) and replace with D5W TKVO. Proper management will also require preload reduction and further investigation as outlined in Chapter 20.

All other forms of shock will require volume expansion. This can be achieved quickly by elevation of the legs (i.e., reverse Trendelenburg's) and administration of repeated small volumes (200 to 300 ml over 15 to 30 min) of an IV fluid that will at least temporarily stay in the intravascular space, e.g., NS and Ringer's lactate.

Reassess volume status after each bolus of IV fluid, aiming for a JVP of 2 to 3 cm H_2O above the sternal angle and concomitant normalization of HR and BP.

If the patient is in *anaphylactic shock* treat rapidly, as follows:

1. IV NS "wide open" until normotensive.
2. *Epinephrine* 0.3 mg (3 ml of a 1:10,000 solution) IV immediately, or 0.3 mg (0.3 ml of a 1:1000 solution) SC immediately with repeat doses q10 to 15 min if indicated. Because the skin is usually hypoperfused during shock, it is better to administer epinephrine IV rather than SC.
3. *Salbutamol* (Ventolin) 2.5 mg/3 ml NS by nebulizer.
4. *Diphenhydramine* (Benadryl) 50 mg IV.
5. *Hydrocortisone* 250 mg IV bolus, followed by 100 mg IV q6h.

Correct hypoxia and acidemia. If the patient is in shock obtain ABGs and administer O_2. If the arterial pH is < 7.2 in the absence of respiratory acidosis, order $NaHCO_3$ 1 amp (44.6 meq) IV. Repeat ABGs every 30 minutes, and repeat $NaHCO_3$ if the patient has not improved.

While restoring the intravascular volume, determine the specific cause of hypotension or shock.

Cardiogenic

This is commonly a result of acute MI. Order stat ECG, portable CXR, and cardiac enzyme tests. However, any of the *CHF etiologic factors* listed on page 207 may be operative.

Be certain the patient is in CHF! Patients with four other conditions can present with hypotension and elevated JVP as follows:

1. *Acute cardiac tamponade* may present with elevated JVP, arterial hypotension, and soft heart sounds (Beck's triad). Suspect this as the diagnosis if there is a pulsus paradoxus of > 10 mm Hg during relaxed respirations (see page 203).
2. A massive *pulmonary embolus* can cause hypotension, elevated JVP, and cyanosis, and may be accompanied by additional evidence of acute right ventricular overload (e.g., positive HJR, RV heave, loud P_2, right-sided S_3, murmur of tricuspid insufficiency).
3. *Superior vena cava obstruction* may present with hypotension and elevated JVP that does not vary with respiration. Additional features may include headache, facial plethora, conjunctival injection, and dilatation of collateral veins on the upper thorax and neck.
4. *Tension pneumothorax* can also cause hypotension and elevated JVP due to positive intrathoracic pressure that decreases venous return to the heart. Look for severe dyspnea, unilateral hyperresonance, and decreased air entry, with tracheal shift *away*

from the involved side. If a tension pneumothorax is suspected, don't wait for x-ray confirmation. Call for your resident and get a #14–16 gauge needle ready to aspirate the pleural space at the second intercostal space in the mid-clavicular line on the affected side. This is a medical emergency!

Hypovolemia

If there is suspicion of a *GI bleed* or another *acute blood loss* being responsible for hypotension, refer to Chapter 10 for further investigation and management.

Excess fluid losses via sweating, vomiting, diarrhea, and polyuria, and *third space losses* (e.g., pancreatitis, peritonitis) will respond to simple intravascular volume expansion with NS or Ringer's lactate and correction of the underlying problem.

Drugs are common causes of hypotension, resulting from relative hypovolemia due to their effects on the heart and peripheral circulation. Common offenders are morphine, meperidine, quinidine, nitroglycerin, beta blockers, calcium entry blockers, captopril, and antihypertensives.

In these instances hypotension is seldom accompanied by evidence of inadequate tissue perfusion and usually can be avoided by reducing the dose or altering the schedule of administration of the drug.

Reverse Trendelenburg's position or a small volume (300 to 500 ml) of NS or Ringer's lactate usually suffices to support the BP until the effect of most drugs wears off. The hypotension of narcotics (morphine, meperidine) can be reversed by *naloxone hydrochloride* (Narcan), 0.2 to 2.0 mg (maximum total dose = 10 mg) IV, SC, or IM, q5 min, until the desired degree of reversal is seen.

Sepsis

Occasionally, intravascular volume repletion and appropriate antibiotics are sufficient to resolve septic shock. Continuing hypotension despite intravascular volume repletion, however, requires ICU/CCU admission for inotropic or vasopressor support.

Anaphylactic Shock

This needs to be recognized and treated immediately to prevent fatal laryngeal edema. Treat as described on page 134.

Remember

1. Consider *toxic shock syndrome* in any hypotensive premenopausal female. Ask about tampon use or, if the patient is obtunded, perform a pelvic examination and remove the tampon, if present.
2. The skin is not a "vital" organ but gives valuable evidence of inadequate tissue perfusion. Remember that during the early

stage of septic shock the skin may be warm and dry owing to abnormal peripheral vasodilatation.
3. Remember that adequate BP is required to perfuse the three vital organs—the *brain, heart,* and *kidney.* After you have successfully rescued your patient from an episode of hypotension look out for "hypotensive sequelae" during the next few days. Not surprisingly, the common sequelae involve these three vital organs:
   a. *Brain.* Thrombotic stroke in a patient with underlying cerebrovascular disease.
   b. *Heart.* MI in a patient with pre-existing atherosclerosis.
   c. *Kidney.* Acute tubular necrosis. Monitor urine output and check urea and creatinine levels in a few days.

Centrilobular hepatic necrosis manifested by jaundice and elevated liver enzymes is also occasionally a sequela of hypotension in the critically ill patient.

16

LINES, TUBES, AND DRAINS

Almost every patient admitted to the hospital will have some form of IV line, tube, or drain inserted during their stay. These devices are useful in the care of patients but, on occasion, will clog, leak, or otherwise malfunction, requiring your expertise and common sense to remedy the problem.

Since the corrective measures that you may have to take when problems arise with lines, tubes, and drains carry the risk of contact with blood and body fluids, make sure you are familiar with and follow your institution's infection control guidelines.

This chapter describes some of the problems that can occur with commonly used lines, tubes, and drains.

CENTRAL LINES

CHEST TUBES

URETHRAL CATHETERS

T-TUBES, J-TUBES, AND PENROSE DRAINS

NASOGASTRIC AND ENTERAL FEEDING TUBES

1. Blocked NG or enteral tube (page 173)
2. Dislodged NG or enteral tube (page 174)

CENTRAL LINES

Blocked Central Lines

Phone Call

Questions

1. **How long has the line been blocked?**
2. **What are the vital signs?**
3. **What was the reason for admission?**

Orders

Ask the RN for a dressing set, two pairs of sterile gloves in your size, chlorhexidine (Hibitane) skin disinfectant, a 5-ml syringe, and a size 20- or 21-gauge needle to be at the bedside. You will probably have to remove the dressing that is securing the central line, and you must keep the site sterile. A second pair of sterile gloves is useful; it is easy to contaminate your gloves when on-call at night.

Inform RN

"Will arrive at the bedside in . . . minutes."

A blocked central line requires you to see the patient immediately.

Elevator Thoughts (What causes a central line to block (Fig. 16–1)?)

1. Kinked tubing
2. Thrombus at the catheter tip

Major Threat to Life

■ Failure of delivery of medications

Interruption in delivery of essential medications may temporarily deprive the patient of required treatment.

Bedside

Quick Look Test

Does the patient look well (comfortable), sick (uncomfortable or distressed), or critical (about to die)?

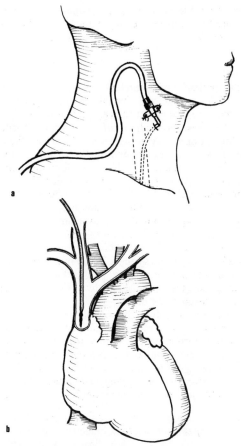

Figure 16–1. Causes of blocked central lines. a = kinked tubing and b = thrombosis at the catheter tip.

A blocked central line, by itself, should not cause the patient to look sick or critical. If the patient looks unwell, search for another cause.

Airway and Vital Signs

A blocked central line should not compromise the airway or other vital signs.

Selective Physical Examination and Management

Inspect the central line. **Is the line kinked?**

If so, remove the dressing securing the line, straighten the line, and now see if there is a flow of IV fluid. If the problem is a kinked line, clean the area using sterile technique and secure the line with a plastic occlusive dressing without re-kinking it.

If there is no flow of IV fluid with the line wide open, proceed as follows:

1. Turn the IV off.
2. Place the patient in Trendelenburg's position (head down). Take the 5-ml syringe and size 20- or 21-gauge capped needle and get ready to disconnect the central line from the IV tubing.
3. During the expiration phase of respiration, disconnect the central line from the IV tubing. Quickly attach the syringe to the central line and the capped needle to the IV tubing. The latter keeps the tubing sterile. The disconnection must be performed quickly to avoid an air embolus. This may result from air being sucked into the line owing to negative intrathoracic pressure generated during inspiration. The risk of an air embolus occurring is diminished by clamping the IV tubing, placing the patient in Trendelenburg's position, and disconnecting the line only during expiration.
4. Draw back gently on the syringe, as too much force will collapse the central line tubing. If the line is blocked with a small thrombus at the distal tip of the line, this maneuver often is sufficient to dislodge the clot.
5. Draw back 3 ml of blood if possible. During the expiratory phase of respiration, remove the capped needle from the end of the IV tubing, remove the syringe from the central line, and re-attach the IV tubing to the central line. Turn the IV on again. Blocked central lines should never be flushed. This maneuver may result in dislodging a clot attached to the catheter tip with subsequent pulmonary embolism.

If the previous maneuvers have been unsuccessful in unblocking the central line, ascertain whether indeed the central line is still necessary. Is the patient receiving medications that can be delivered only via a central line (e.g., amphotericin, dopamine, nitroglycerin, TPN)? Was the central line started because of lack of peripheral vein access? If so, re-examine the patient to see if there are now any peripheral veins suitable for IV access.

If central venous access is essential, the next step is to insert a new central line at a different site. A new central line should not be inserted over a guidewire placed through the blocked central line, since the insertion of the guidewire may also dislodge a clot.

In situations where central venous access is essential, and no alternative sites are available, streptokinase and urokinase have been used to dissolve the obstructing clot. Significant risks are involved with the use of these agents, and hence routine use is not recommended.

Bleeding at the Central Line Entry Site

Phone Call

Questions

1. **What are the vital signs?**
2. **What was the reason for admission?**

Orders
Ask for a dressing set, two pairs of sterile gloves in your size, and chlorhexidine (Hibitane) skin disinfectant to be at the bedside. You will probably have to remove the plastic occlusive dressing that is securing the central line, and you must keep the site sterile.

Inform RN
"Will arrive at the bedside in . . . minutes."
Bleeding at the central line site requires you to see the patient immediately.

Elevator Thoughts (What causes bleeding at the line insertion site?)

1. Oozing of subcutaneous and cutaneous blood vessels (capillaries)
2. Coagulation disorders
   a. Drugs (warfarin, heparin, aspirin, NSAIDs)
   b. Thrombocytopenia, platelet dysfunction
   c. Clotting factor deficiency

Major Threat to Life

■ Upper airway obstruction

Bleeding into the soft tissues of the neck may cause tracheal compression resulting in life-threatening upper airway obstruction. The patient may look sick or critical if excessive blood loss has occurred.

Bedside

Quick Look Test
Does the patient look well (comfortable), sick (uncomfortable or distressed), or critical (about to die)?
These patients look well unless there is an upper airway obstruction.

Airway and Vital Signs

Check the airway. **What is the RR?**

If there is any evidence of an upper airway obstruction (inspiratory stridor or significant soft tissue swelling of the neck), call the ICU/CCU team immediately.

Selective Physical Examination and Management

1. Remove the dressing and try to identify a specific area of bleeding.
2. If you are unable to identify a specific site of bleeding, clean the site using sterile technique and reinspect the area. Usually, general oozing of blood is seen at the entry site, with no one specific skin vessel identified as the culprit.
3. Apply continuous pressure to the entry site for the next 20 minutes. This is performed by applying, with a gloved hand, a folded, sterile 2-cm × 2-cm gauze dressing to the site with firm, continuous pressure. Do not release this pressure during the 20 minutes since the platelet plug you are allowing to form will be broken (see Fig. 16–2).
4. Re-inspect the entry site. If the bleeding has stopped, clean the area using sterile technique and secure the line with plastic occlusive dressing. If there is still bleeding at the site, then repeat the previous maneuver for another 20 minutes. Provided *continuous* pressure has been applied, any bleeding should have stopped. In the unusual circumstance where bleeding has not stopped, a coagulation disorder should be suspected. Refer to Chapter 25 for management of coagulation problems. Alternatively, a single suture may be placed at the site of bleeding, in an attempt to provide hemostasis.
5. Removal of the central line should be considered if bleeding at the insertion site is excessive and resistant to the previous measures.

Shortness of Breath Following Central Line Insertion

Phone Call

Questions

1. **How long has the patient been SOB?**
2. **What are the vital signs?**
3. **What was the reason for admission?**

Orders

1. Ask the RN for a dressing set, two pairs of sterile gloves in your size, chlorhexidine (Hibitane) skin disinfectant, and a size 16 IV catheter to be at the bedside. If the patient has a tension pneumothorax you will need to insert a size 16 IV catheter into

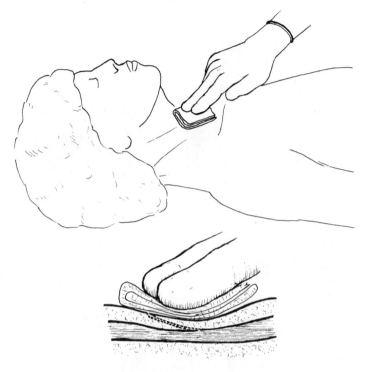

Figure 16–2. Continuous firm local pressure is required for 20 min to stop the oozing of blood from the central line entry site. Make sure the pressure is applied over the puncture site in the vein and not at the skin entry site.

    the second intercostal space on the hyperresonant side, with your resident's guidance.
2. If you suspect a pneumothorax, order a stat portable CXR in the upright position in expiration. Hypotension, tachypnea, and pleuritic chest pain after central line insertion are suggestive of a pneumothorax.
3. Order O_2 by mask at 10 L/min.

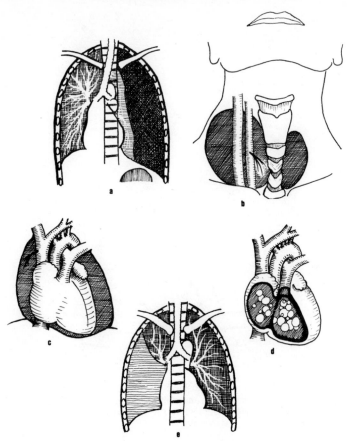

Figure 16–3. Causes of SOB following central line insertion. a = pneumothorax, b = massive soft tissue hematoma from inadvertent carotid artery puncture resulting in upper airway obstruction, c = cardiac tamponade, d = air embolus, and e = pleural effusion.

Inform RN

"Will arrive at the bedside in . . . minutes."

SOB after central line insertion requires you to see the patient immediately.

Elevator Thoughts (What causes shortness of breath following central line insertion (Fig. 16–3)?)

- Pneumothorax
- Massive soft tissue hematoma from inadvertent carotid artery puncture, resulting in upper airway obstruction

- Cardiac tamponade
- Air embolus
- Pleural effusion

Major Threat to Life

- Pneumothorax
- Cardiac tamponade
- Upper airway obstruction
- Air embolus

A tension pneumothorax may develop minutes to days after the insertion of a central line, if pleural perforation occurred during insertion. Rarely, cardiac tamponade results from perforation by the catheter of the right atrium or right ventricle. Upper airway obstruction may result from a massive soft tissue hematoma (e.g., from an inadvertent carotid artery puncture). Air may be inadvertently introduced if the line is disconnected incorrectly.

Bedside

Quick Look Test

Does the patient look well (comfortable), sick (uncomfortable or distressed), or critical (about to die)?

A patient with pneumothorax or upper airway obstruction looks sick or critical.

Airway and Vital Signs

Check the airway. If there is any evidence of an upper airway obstruction (i.e., inspiratory stridor or significant soft tissue swelling of the neck) call the ICU/CCU team immediately.

What are the BP and RR?

Hypotension and tachypnea in a patient with a recently inserted central line may indicate a tension pneumothorax or cardiac tamponade, inadvertently caused at the time of line insertion. See page 134 for the assessment and page 146 for the management of tension pneumothorax and cardiac tamponade.

Selective Physical Examination

RESP   Tracheal deviation (pneumothorax)
                         Unilateral hyperresonance to percussion (pneumothorax)
                         Stony dullness to percussion, decreased breath sounds, decreased tactile fremitus (pleural effusion)

CVS   Pulsus paradoxus (cardiac tamponade)
                         Pulsus paradoxus is present when the de-

crease in systolic BP with inspiration is >
10 mm Hg. (The normal variation in systolic
BP in quiet respiration is 0 to 10 mm Hg).
A pulsus paradoxus is definitely present if
the radial pulse disappears during inspiration.
Kussmaul's sign (occasionally seen in cardiac
tamponade)
Kussmaul's sign is an increase in the JVP
during inspiration
Elevated JVP (cardiac tamponade)
Distant heart sounds (pericardial effusion or
cardiac tamponade (COPD)

CENTRAL LINE   Check all IV connections to ensure they are
not loose (air embolus)

Management

Tension pneumothorax is a medical emergency requiring urgent
treatment. You will need supervision by your resident or attending
physician.

1. Identify the second intercostal space in the mid-clavicular line
   on the affected (hyperresonant) side.
2. Mark this point with the pressure from a capped needle or ball-
   point pen.
3. Open the dressing set and pour the chlorhexidine (Hibitane)
   into the appropriate space.
4. Put on the sterile gloves.
5. Clean the area identified previously.
6. Insert the size 16 IV catheter into the designated area. If a
   tension pneumothorax is present there will be a loud sound of
   air rushing out through the catheter. You will not need to
   connect the catheter to suction, since the lung will decompress
   itself.
7. Order a chest tube sent to the room immediately. The definitive
   treatment is the insertion of a chest tube.

Small pneumothoraces usually undergo spontaneous reabsorption
over a few days.

Large or symptomatic pneumothoraces require chest tube drainage.

Cardiac tamponade is a medical emergency.

1. Clamp the IV tubing and turn off the IV.
2. Call the ICU/CCU team immediately for possible urgent peri-
   cardiocentesis.
3. Volume expansion with NS, through a large bore IV, may be a
   useful temporizing measure to help maintain adequate CO.

Massive unilateral pleural effusion should be managed as follows:

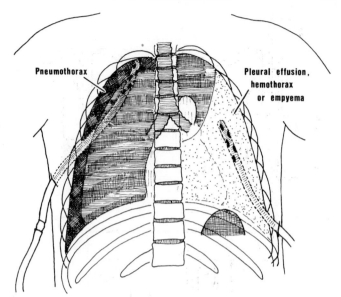

Pneumothorax

Pleural effusion,
hemothorax
or empyema

Figure 16–4. Chest tubes are inserted to drain air (pneumothoraces), blood (hemothoraces), fluid (pleural effusions), and pus (empyemas).

1. Clamp the IV tubing and stop the IV fluid.
2. Thoracentesis will be required if the patient is markedly SOB.

Air embolism may be helped by placing the patient on the right side in Trendelenburg's position (head down), in order to trap the air bubbles in the right ventricle and prevent them from entering the pulmonary artery. The patient should be kept in this position until the air bubbles have been reabsorbed. (Aspiration of air bubbles from the right ventricle is advocated by some experts.) Re-inspect all the IV connections and make certain they are secure. If necessary a new central line may have to be inserted.

CHEST TUBES

Chest tubes are inserted to drain air (pneumothoraces), blood (hemothoraces), fluid (pleural effusions), or pus (empyemas) (Fig. 16–4). They should always be connected to an underwater seal; they may be left to straight drainage (no suction), or more commonly, to suction. Figure 16–5 illustrates the various chest tube drainage apparatuses. Common chest tube problems are illustrated in Figure 16–6.

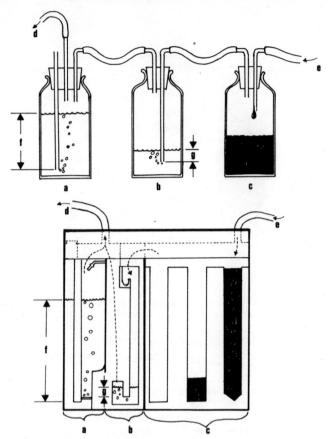

Figure 16–5. Chest tube apparatuses. a = suction control chamber, b = underwater seal, c = collection chamber, d = to suction, e = from patient, f = height equals amount of suction in cm H_2O, and g = height equals underwater seal in cm H_2O.

Persistent Bubbling in the Drainage Container("Air Leak")

Phone Call

Questions

1. Why was the chest tube inserted?
2. What are the vital signs?
3. Is the patient SOB?
4. What was the reason for admission?

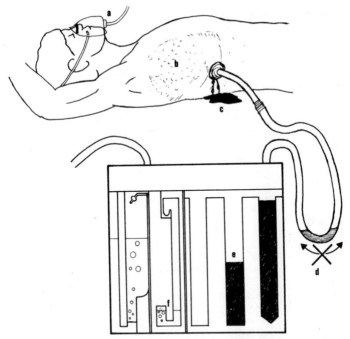

Figure 16–6. Common chest tube problems. a = SOB, b = subcutaneous emphysema, c = bleeding at the entry site, d = loss of fluctuation, e = excessive drainage, and f = persistent bubbling.

Orders
    Nil

Inform the RN
    "Will arrive at the bedside in . . . minutes."
    Persistent bubbling in the drainage container is a potential emergency, requiring you to see the patient as soon as possible. Any malfunctioning of the chest tube, if associated with SOB, requires you to see the patient immediately.

Elevator Thoughts (What causes persistent bubbling in the drainage compartment?)

1. Loose tubing connection
2. Traumatic tracheobronchial injury. A large, persistent air leak in traumatic pneumothorax suggests a concomitant tracheobronchial injury.
3. Persistent bronchopleural air leak

  a. Post-lobectomy
  b. Ruptured bleb or bulla (e.g., asthma, emphysema)
  c. Following intrathoracic procedures (e.g., needle biopsy, thoracentesis)

Major Threat to Life

A persistent "air leak" suggests either a pneumothorax from intrathoracic injury or a loose connection of the drainage apparatus. Hence, the major threat to life is the underlying intrathoracic disease process responsible for the persistent air leak. As long as air continues to bubble through the collection chamber, one can be reasonably certain that excessive intrapleural air will not accumulate.

Bedside

Quick Look Test
Does the patient look well (comfortable), sick (uncomfortable or distressed), or critical (about to die)?

If a small air leak is the problem, the patient may look well. A patient who looks sick may be developing a larger pneumothorax or may look sick for unrelated reasons.

Airway and Vital Signs

Provided all tubing connections are snug, a persistent air leak means that the patient has a pneumothorax. As long as air continues to bubble through the collection chamber, the pneumothorax should drain and thus not result in alteration of vital signs.

Selective History and Chart Review
Why was the chest tube inserted?

If the chest tube was inserted to drain a pneumothorax, the tube should be bubbling, unless the lung is fully expanded and the leak has sealed.

If the chest tube was inserted to drain a hemothorax, a pleural effusion, or an empyema with straight drainage (no suction), then new onset of bubbling in the collection chamber represents either loose tubing connections or development of a pneumothorax.

Selective Physical Examination and Management

Provided a pneumothorax is not present, a persistent air leak is indicated by air bubbles in the underwater seal section of the Pleur-evac while the suction is turned off. If the air leak is small it may be seen only with measures that increase intrapleural pressure (e.g., coughing) (see Fig. 16–6).

Clamp the chest tube as close to the patient as possible, without removing the dressing, and observe the underwater seal chamber for any air bubbles. Next, clamp the chest tube as close to the Pleur-evac or drainage bottles as possible, and again observe the underwater seal chamber for any air bubbles.

Air bubbles stopped by clamping the tube at both sites will indicate a persistent pneumothorax. Order a stat upright portable CXR (in expiration) to ascertain whether the chest tube is adequately positioned to allow drainage of the pneumothorax.

Remove the dressing at the entry site of the chest tube, listen for "sucking sounds," and observe the incision area. If the incision is too large and inadequately closed, insert one to two sterile 2–0 sutures to seal the opening. If the incision is adequately closed with sutures, re-apply a pressure dressing ensuring that the Vaseline (petrolatum) gauze occlusive dressing seals the incision.

Air bubbles not stopped by clamping the tube either proximally or distally indicate an air leak in the Pleur-evac or drainage apparatus or a leak around the chest tube entry site. Alternatively, the chest tube may have been dislodged, and one of the drainage apertures may be outside the chest wall. Ensure that the connections are tight. If this does not correct the bubbling, a new Pleur-evac or other drainage apparatus should be used.

If air bubbles are stopped by clamping the tube distally but not proximally, the leak is in the tubing itself or at the connection between the chest tube and the connecting tubing; re-tape the connection. If this does not stop the leak, new connecting tubing will be required.

Remember to unclamp the chest tube. *Never leave a patient with a clamped chest tube unattended;* a tension pneumothorax may develop rapidly if a ball-valve mechanism is present.

Bleeding Around the Chest Tube Entry Site

Phone Call

Questions

1. **Why was the chest tube inserted?**
2. **What are the vital signs?**
3. **Is the patient SOB?**
4. **What was the reason for admission?**

Orders
Ask the RN for a dressing set, two pairs of sterile gloves in your size, and chlorhexidine (Hibitane) skin cleanser to be at the bedside. You will have to remove the dressing around the chest tube, and you must keep the site sterile.

Inform RN
"Will arrive at the bedside in . . . minutes."

Bleeding around the chest tube entry site is a potential emergency, requiring you to see the patient as soon as possible. Any malfunctioning chest tube in association with SOB requires you to see the patient immediately.

Elevator Thoughts (What causes bleeding around the chest tube entry site?)

1. Inadequate pressure bandage
2. Inadequate closure of the incision with the suture
3. Coagulation disorders
4. Trauma to intercostal vessels or lung during insertion of the chest tube
5. Blockage of chest tube or inadequate sized chest tube with drainage of the hemothorax around the entry site

Major Threat to Life

■ Hemorrhagic shock

Continuous oozing, if allowed to progress, may eventually lead to intravascular depletion and, in the extreme case, hemorrhagic shock.

Bedside

Quick Look Test
Does the patient look well (comfortable), sick (uncomfortable or distressed), or critical (about to die)?
If there is only a small amount of bleeding from the chest tube entry site, the patient will probably look entirely well. A patient who has lost more blood may look sick or critical.

Airway and Vital Signs
What are the BP and RR?
Hypotension and tachycardia may indicate major loss of blood. Tachypnea may indicate a large hemothorax.

Selective History and Chart Review

1. Why was the chest tube inserted?
2. Check the following recent laboratory results: Hb, PT, aPTT, and platelet count

Selective Physical Examination and Management

Remove the dressing at the chest tube entry site and inspect the incision. If the incision is too large and inadequately closed, insert one or two sutures to seal the opening. If the incision is adequately closed with the sutures, re-apply a pressure dressing over the site taking care to ensure the pressure is maintained. The aforementioned maneuvers when performed adequately will stop the bleeding in the majority of situations.

Is the chest tube obstructed, resulting in blood draining around the entry site? Try "milking" the chest tube. Re-inspect to see if this maneuver re-established fluctuation in the underwater seal. The connecting tubing is made of rubber and may be carefully "stripped" using the chest tube strippers. These two maneuvers help dislodge blood clots and debris that may be blocking the tube.

Is the chest tube too small, thus unable to drain a large hemothorax adequately? A larger size chest tube may be required.

Drainage of an Excessive Volume of Blood

Phone Call

Questions

1. **Why was the chest tube inserted?**
2. **What are the vital signs?**
3. **Is the patient SOB?**
4. **What was the reason for admission?**

Orders
   Nil

Inform RN
   "Will arrive at the bedside in . . . minutes."

Drainage of an excessive volume of blood via the chest tube is a potential emergency and requires you to see the patient immediately. Any malfunctioning chest tube, when in association with SOB, requires you to see the patient immediately.

Elevator Thoughts (What causes excessive blood to drain via the chest tube?)

Intrathoracic bleeding

Major Threat to Life

■ Hemorrhagic shock

Hemorrhagic shock may result from excessive intrathoracic blood loss.

Bedside

Quick Look Test
   Does the patient look well (comfortable), sick (uncomfortable or distressed), or critical (about to die)?

A patient with hemorrhagic shock will look pale, sweaty, and restless.

Airway and Vital Signs
What are the BP and HR?
Hypotension and tachycardia may indicate hemorrhagic shock.
What is the RR?
Tachypnea and hypotension may indicate a tension pneumothorax.

Management I

1. If the patient is hypotensive, draw 20 ml of blood and start a large bore IV (#16 if possible). Give 500 ml of NS or Ringer's lactate IV as fast as possible.
2. Send blood for an immediate crossmatch for 4 to 6 units of packed RBCs on hold; Hb, PT, aPTT, and platelet count; plus electrolyte, creatinine, and glucose levels.

Selective Chart Review and Management
Is the patient receiving anticoagulant medication (heparin, warfarin)?
If so, review the initial indication for anticoagulation. Can the anticoagulants be safely discontinued or reversed? Consult hematology for assistance in the management of this difficult and potentially life-threatening situation.

Estimate how much blood the patient has lost over the past 48 hours by reviewing the intake/output chart.
If the patient has lost more than 500 ml over 8 hours: Consultation with a thoracic surgeon is recommended. The patient may need immediate transfer to the operating room for an emergency thoracotomy.

If the patient has lost less than 500 ml over 8 hours: Order hourly monitoring of the blood lost via the chest tube, noting that a physician needs to be informed if the blood loss is greater than 50 ml/hr.

Loss of Fluctuation of the Underwater Seal

Phone Call

Questions

1. **Why was the chest tube inserted?**
2. **What are the vital signs?**
3. **Is the patient SOB?**
4. **What was the reason for admission?**

Orders
Nil

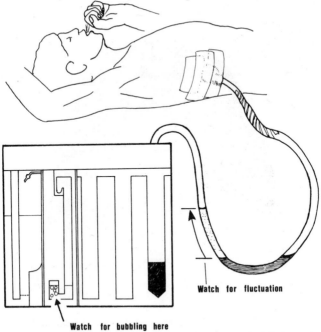

Figure 16–7. Loss of fluctuation of the underwater seal. Ask the patient to cough, and observe for any fluctuation or bubbling.

Inform RN

"Will arrive at the bedside in . . . minutes."

Loss of fluctuation of the underwater seal is a potential emergency and requires you to see the patient as soon as possible. Any malfunctioning chest tube, when associated with SOB, requires you to see the patient immediately.

Elevator Thoughts (What causes loss of fluctuation of the underwater seal?)

1. Kinked chest tube
2. Plugged chest tube
3. Improper chest tube positioning

The underwater seal is essentially a one-way, low resistance valve. During expiration the intrapleural pressure increases, becoming higher than atmospheric pressure, forcing air or fluid that is in the pleural space through the chest tube and underwater seal (Fig. 16–7).

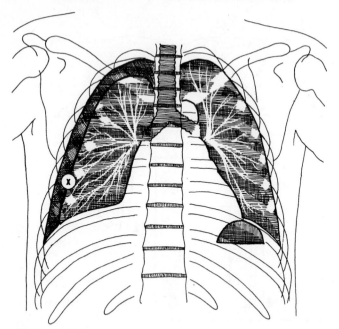

Figure 16–8. Pneumothorax. x = edge of visceral pleura or lung.

Major Threat to Life

- Tension pneumothorax

Inadequate drainage of a pneumothorax by a blocked chest tube may lead to a tension pneumothorax (Fig. 16–8 and Fig. 16–9).

Bedside

Quick Look Test
Does the patient look well (comfortable), sick (uncomfortable or distressed), or critical (about to die)?
A patient who looks sick may be developing a tension pneumothorax or may look sick for unrelated reasons.

Airway and Vital Signs
What are the BP and RR?
Hypotension and tachypnea may indicate a tension pneumothorax.

Selective History and Chart Review

1. Why was the chest tube inserted?

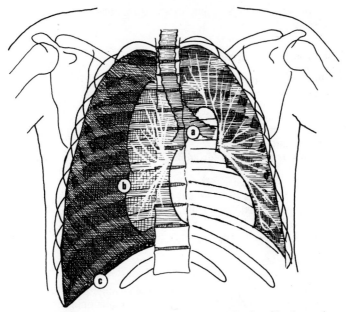

Figure 16–9. Tension pneumothorax. a = shifted mediastinum, b = edge of collapsed lung, and c = low flattened diaphragm.

2. How long ago did the chest tube stop fluctuating?
3. What has been draining from the chest tube? What volume has drained over the past 24 hours?

Selective Physical Examination and Management

1. Inspect the underwater seal. Is there any fluctuation? Ask the patient to cough and observe the tube for any fluctuation. A chest tube with its distal aperture located within the pleural space fluctuates with respiration.
2. Inspect the chest tube for kinking. You may need to remove the dressing at the chest tube site. If the chest tube is kinked, reposition and reinspect it for fluctuation of the underwater seal.
3. Try "milking" the chest tube. Re-inspect to see if this maneuver re-establishes fluctuation in the underwater seal. The connecting tubing is rubber and may be carefully stripped using chest tube strippers. These two maneuvers help dislodge blood clots and debris that may be blocking the tube.
4. Order a portable CXR. Improper positioning of the chest tube may result in a loss of fluctuation of the underwater seal.
5. If the tube is not fluctuating after all the aforementioned

maneuvers are attempted, a new chest tube may have to be inserted.

Subcutaneous Emphysema

Phone Call

Questions

1. **Why was the chest tube inserted?**
2. **What are the vital signs?**
3. **Is the patient SOB?**
4. **What was the reason for admission?**

Orders

Ask the RN for a dressing set, two pairs of sterile gloves in your size, and chlorhexidine (Hibitane) skin cleanser to be at the bedside. You will have to remove the dressing around the chest tube, and you must keep the site sterile.

Inform RN

"Will arrive at the bedside in . . . minutes."

Subcutaneous emphysema is a potential emergency requiring you to see the patient immediately. Any malfunctioning chest tube, if associated with SOB, requires you to see the patient immediately.

Elevator Thoughts (What causes subcutaneous emphysema?)

1. Chest tube may be too small for the size of the leak
2. Inadequate suction
3. One of the chest tube apertures may be in the chest wall.
4. Chest tube may be in the chest wall or abdominal cavity.
5. Insignificant localized subcutaneous emphysema around the entry site is not uncommon after chest tube insertion.

Major Threat to Life

■ Upper airway obstruction

If subcutaneous emphysema extends up into the neck, there may be tracheal compression resulting in upper airway obstruction.

Bedside

Quick Look Test

Does the patient look well (comfortable), sick (uncomfortable or distressed), or critical (about to die)?

The patient with upper airway obstruction will look sick or critical, and there may be audible inspiratory stridor.

Airway and Vital Signs

1. Inspect and palpate the neck for SC emphysema.
2. **What is the RR?** The patient with upper airway obstruction will have tachypnea.
3. **What are the BP and HR?** SC emphysema may be accompanied by a tension pneumothorax. If so, the patient will have a tachycardia.

Selective History and Chart Review
Why was the chest tube inserted?

Selective Physical Examination and Management

1. If there is significant upper airway obstruction (palpable SC emphysema over the trachea, inspiratory stridor, tachypnea) call the ICU/CCU team immediately for probable intubation and transfer to the ICU/CCU. Cardiothoracic surgery may be required if mediastinal decompression is indicated.
2. **What size chest tube has been inserted? Is the chest tube too small in diameter?** Multi-fenestrated vinyl chest tubes are available in the two following sizes: 20F and 36F. The 20F may not be large enough, and air may escape from the pleural cavity into the chest wall, resulting in SC emphysema. If the chest tube is too small, a larger one will need to be inserted. Sometimes two large chest tubes may be required for adequate drainage.
3. **Is the chest tube connected to suction?** A large pneumothorax may not be adequately drained if it is connected only to an underwater seal, as opposed to suction.
4. Remove the dressing at the chest tube site and inspect the chest tube. **Are any of the drainage holes in the distal end of the chest tube visible?** None of the drainage lines should be visible; they should all be inside the pleural cavity. SC emphysema may be caused by misplacement of the chest tube, with one of the drainage holes inadvertently in the soft tissues of the chest wall. A new chest tube should be inserted. Do not re-introduce the partially extruded chest tube since you may introduce infection into the pleural space.

Shortness of Breath

Phone Call

Questions

1. **Why was the chest tube inserted?**
2. **What are the vital signs?**
3. **What was the reason for admission?**

Orders

Ask the RN for a dressing set, two pairs of sterile gloves in your size, chlorhexidine (Hibitane) skin cleanser, and a size 16 IV catheter. A tension pneumothorax, if present, is most effectively treated with insertion of a size 16 IV catheter into the pleural space on the affected side.

Inform RN

"Will arrive at the bedside in . . . minutes."

SOB in a patient with a chest tube in place is a potential emergency and requires you to see the patient immediately.

Elevator Thoughts (What causes shortness of breath in a patient with a chest tube?)

Causes Related to the Chest Tube

1. Tension pneumothorax
2. Increasing pneumothorax. Both 1 and 2 may occur with
   a. Inadequate suction
   b. Misplaced tube (i.e., chest tube not in the pleural cavity)
   c. Blocked or kinked tube
   d. Bronchopulmonary fistula
3. Subcutaneous emphysema
4. Increasing pleural effusion or hemothorax
5. Re-expansion pulmonary edema (Sometimes this occurs after rapid expansion of a pneumothorax, drainage of pleural fluid, or both.)

Causes Unrelated to the Chest Tube

See Chapter 20, page 200.

Major Threat to Life

- Tension pneumothorax
- Upper airway obstruction

Inadequate drainage of a pneumothorax produced through a ball-valve mechanism may result in a life-threatening tension pneumothorax. Tracheal compression from interstitial emphysema may cause upper airway obstruction.

Bedside

Quick Look Test

Does the patient look well (comfortable), sick (uncomfortable or distressed), or critical (about to die)?

A sick or critical looking patient may have a tension pneumothorax or may have an unrelated reason for SOB (see Chapter 20).

Airway and Vital Signs

1. Inspect and palpate the neck for SC emphysema.
2. **What is the RR?** Rates > 20/min suggest hypoxia, pain, or anxiety. Look for thoracoabdominal dissociation which may indicate impending respiratory failure. Remember that the rib cage and abdominal wall normally move in the same direction during inspiration and expiration.
3. **What are the BP and HR?** Hypotension and tachycardia may indicate a tension pneumothorax or another unrelated cause of SOB (see Chapter 20).

Selective Physical Examination
Does the patient have a tension pneumothorax?

VITALS	Tachypnea
	Hypotension
HEENT	Tracheal deviation away from the hyperresonant side
RESP	Unilateral hyperresonance
	Decreased air entry on hyperresonant side
CVS	Elevated JVP
CHEST TUBE	Is there bubbling in the collection chamber?
	Absence of bubbling suggests malposition or malfunction of the chest tube.

Selective Chart Review
Why was the chest tube inserted?

Management

1. If there is *significant upper airway obstruction* (palpable subcutaneous emphysema over the trachea, inspiratory stridor, tachypnea) call the ICU/CCU team immediately for probable intubation and transfer to the ICU/CCU.
2. *Tension pneumothorax* is a medical emergency requiring urgent treatment. You will need supervision by your resident or attending physician.
   a. Identify the second intercostal space in the mid-clavicular line on the affected (hyperresonant) side.
   b. Mark this point using pressure from the cap of a needle or ball-point pen.
   c. Open the dressing set and pour the chlorhexidine (Hibitane) into the appropriate container.
   d. Put on the sterile gloves.
   e. Clean the area previously identified.
   f. Insert the size 16 IV catheter into the designated area. If a tension pneumothorax is present there will be a loud sound of air rushing out through the catheter. You will not need

to connect the catheter to suction, since the pleural space will decompress itself.

   g. Order a chest tube sent to the room immediately. The definitive treatment is the insertion of a chest tube.

3. If there is an *increasing pneumothorax* but no evidence of a tension pneumothorax order a stat upright CXR in expiration. Meanwhile, look for any correctable causes, e.g., kinked or blocked tubing, inadequate suction, and dislodged chest tube.

4. For the management of other causes of SOB, i.e., causes unrelated to chest tubes, see Chapter 20.

URETHRAL CATHETERS

There are five types of urethral catheters (Fig. 16–10). *Foley's* (balloon retention) *catheter* is the most commonly used of these; it consists of a double lumen tube; the larger lumen drains urine, and the smaller lumen admits 5 to 30 ml of water to inflate the balloon tip. *Straight (Robinson's) catheters* are used to obtain in-out collections of urine, to obtain sterile specimens in patients who are unable to void voluntarily, and to obtain post-voiding residual urine volume measurements. A *coudé catheter* has a curved tip that facilitates insertion when a urethral obstruction (e.g., benign prostatic hypertrophy) makes passage of Foley's catheter difficult. *Three-way irrigation catheters* have, in addition to lumens for urine drainage and balloon inflation, a third lumen for bladder irrigation. These catheters are commonly used after transurethral prostate resection to facilitate bladder irrigation and drainage of blood clots. A *Silastic catheter* is similar to Foley's catheter, but is constructed of softer, less reactive plastic; it is used when a urethral catheter is required on a long-term basis.

Blocked Urethral Catheter

Phone Call

Questions

1. **How long has the catheter been blocked?**
2. **What are the vital signs?**
3. **Does the patient have suprapubic pain?**
   Urinary retention secondary to a blocked catheter can result in suprapubic pain due to bladder distention.
4. **What was the reason for admission?**

Orders
Ask the RN to try flushing the catheter with 30 to 40 ml of sterile NS, if this has not been done.

Inform RN

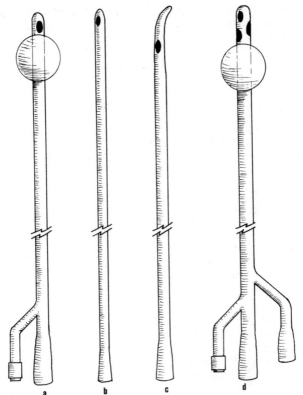

Figure 16–10. Urethral catheters. a = Foley's catheter, b = straight (Robinson's) catheter, c = coudé catheter, and d = three-way irrigation catheter.

"Will arrive at the bedside in . . . minutes."

Provided the patient does not have suprapubic pain (bladder distention), assessment of a blocked urinary catheter can wait an hour or two if other problems of higher priority exist.

Elevator Thoughts (What causes blocked urethral catheters?)

1. Urinary sediment
2. Blood clots
3. Kinked catheter (look under the bedsheets!)
4. Improperly placed or dislodged catheter

Major Threat to Life

■ Bladder rupture
■ Progressive renal insufficiency

Bladder rupture may occur if bladder distention progresses without decompression. Since bladder distention is painful, bladder rupture from this cause usually is seen only in the unconscious or paraplegic patient. Persistent lower urinary tract obstruction may lead to hydronephrosis and renal failure.

Bedside

Quick Look Test

Does the patient look well (comfortable), sick (uncomfortable or distressed), or critical (about to die)?

Most patients with blocked urethral catheters look well. However, patients with acute bladder distention may look distressed because of abdominal pain.

Airway and Vital Signs

A blocked urethral catheter is not usually responsible for alterations in vital signs unless pain due to bladder distention causes tachypnea or tachycardia.

Selective Physical Examination and Management

1. Percuss and palpate the abdomen to determine whether the bladder is distended. Suprapubic dullness and tenderness suggest a distended bladder.
2. Examine the tubing for kinking of the catheter, blood clots, or sediment.
3. Order a sterile dressing tray, a 50-ml bulb syringe (or a 50-ml syringe and an adapter), and two pairs of sterile gloves in your size. Aspirate and irrigate the catheter with 30 to 40 ml of sterile NS as follows:
   a. Ask an assistant to hold the distal part of the catheter close to the connection between the tubing and urinary drainage bag.
   b. Wear sterile gloves and clean the distal catheter and the proximal connecting tubing with chlorhexidine.
   c. Disconnect the drainage tubing from the catheter. Ask an assistant to hold the connecting tubing in the air to maintain a sterile tip.
   d. Using a 50-ml syringe, aspirate the catheter vigorously to dislodge and extract any blood clots or sediment that may have blocked the catheter. If the maneuver is unsuccessful, flush the catheter with 30 to 40 ml of sterile NS. Several attempts at aspiration should be made before abandoning this technique.
   e. Reconnect the catheter to the connecting tubing, ensuring sterile technique.
   The majority of blocked Foley's catheters will become unplugged with this maneuver.

4. If flushing of the catheter fails to relieve obstruction, a new catheter should be inserted if one is still required.

Gross Hematuria

Phone Call

Questions

1. **Why was the urethral catheter inserted?**
2. **What are the vital signs?**
3. **Is the patient receiving anticoagulant drugs or cyclophosphamide?**
4. **What was the reason for admission?**

Orders
Nil

Inform RN
"Will arrive at the bedside in . . . minutes."

Gross hematuria in the anticoagulated patient requires you to see the patient immediately.

Elevator Thoughts (What causes gross hematuria in the catheterized patient?)

Urethral Trauma

- Inadvertent or partial removal of the catheter with the balloon still inflated
- During catheter insertion

Drugs

- Anticoagulants (heparin, warfarin)
- Cyclophosphamide

Coagulation Abnormalities

- DIC
- Specific factor deficiencies
- Thrombocytopenia

Unrelated Problems

- Renal stones
- Carcinoma of the kidney, bladder, or prostate
- Glomerulonephritis
- Prostatitis
- Rupture of a bladder vein

Major Threat to Life

- Hemorrhagic shock

Although gross hematuria is dramatic and most distressing to the patient, it is quite rare for bleeding to be significant enough to result in hemorrhagic shock. It only requires 1 ml of blood in 1 L of urine to change the color from yellow to red.

Bedside

Quick Look Test
Does the patient look well (comfortable), sick (uncomfortable or distressed), or critical (about to die)?

It is unusual for these patients to look other than well. If they look sick or critical, search for a separate unrecognized problem.

Airway and Vital Signs
What is the BP?

Hypotension in the patient with gross hematuria may be a sign of hemorrhagic shock.

What is the HR?

A resting tachycardia, though a non-specific finding, may indicate hypovolemia if significant blood loss has occurred.

Selective History and Chart Review
Is the patient receiving any of the following medications?

- Heparin, warfarin
- Cyclophosphamide

Is there any abnormality in the coagulation profile?

- PT, aPTT, platelet count

Is there any history of urethral trauma?

- Recent inadvertent removal of Foley's catheter with the balloon still inflated (especially in the elderly, confused patient)
- Recent GU surgery
- Recent difficulty with insertion of a urethral catheter

Has there been a recent decrease in the Hb value? How much blood has the patient lost?

- Bleeding via the urinary tract is unlikely to cause significant hemodynamic changes unless there has been recent GU surgery.

Management

1. If the patient is anticoagulated, review the initial indication for the anticoagulation. Decide, in consultation with your resident

and a hematologist, whether the risk of anticoagulation is still warranted.

2. If a coagulation abnormality is identified refer to Chapter 25 for discussion of the investigation and management.

3. If there is a history of recent urethral trauma, continued significant blood loss is unlikely. Have the vital signs taken every 4 to 6 hours for the next 24 hours. Significant bleeding may be manifested by tachycardia and orthostatic hypotension.

Inability to Insert a Urethral Catheter

Phone Call

Questions

1. **Why was the urethral catheter ordered?**
2. **What are the vital signs?**
3. **Does the patient have suprapubic pain?**
4. **How many attempts have been made to catheterize the patient?**
5. **What was the reason for admission?**

Orders

Ask the RN for a catheter insertion set, two pairs of sterile gloves in your size, and chlorhexidine (Hibitane) skin disinfectant to be at the bedside.

Inform RN

"Will arrive at the bedside in . . . minutes."

Provided the patient does not have suprapubic pain (bladder distention), insertion of a urethral catheter can wait an hour or two if other problems of higher priority exist.

Elevator Thoughts (What causes difficulty in urethral catheterization?)

Urethral Edema

■ Multiple insertion attempts
■ Inadvertent removal of a Foley's catheter with the balloon still inflated

Urethral Obstruction

■ Benign prostatic hypertrophy
■ Carcinoma of the prostate
■ Urethral stricture
■ Anatomic anomaly (diverticulum, false passage)

Major Threat to Life

■ Bladder rupture
■ Progressive renal insufficiency

Bladder rupture may occur if bladder distention is not relieved by the placement of a urinary catheter. A suprapubic catheter may be required if urethral catheterization is impossible. Persistent bladder obstruction may lead to hydronephrosis and renal failure.

Bedside

Quick Look Test

Does the patient look well (comfortable), sick (uncomfortable or distressed), or critical (about to die)?

Patients with acute bladder distention may look distressed because of abdominal pain.

Airway and Vital Signs

Inability to insert a urethral catheter should not compromise the vital signs.

Selective History and Chart Review

1. **Is there a history of recent, multiple attempts at catheterization or removal of a catheter with the balloon still inflated (urethral edema)?**
2. **Is there a history of a benign prostatic hypertrophy, carcinoma of the prostate, urethral stricture, or an anatomic abnormality of the urethra?**
3. **What was the original indication for urethral catheter placement? Does the indication still exist?**

Selective Physical Examination and Management

1. Percuss and palpate the abdomen to determine whether the bladder is distended. Suprapubic dullness and tenderness are suggestive of a distended bladder.
2. If urethral edema is suspected, try inserting a smaller sized catheter.
3. If there is a history of urethral obstruction, try inserting a coudé catheter.
4. If you are unable to catheterize the patient, consult urology for assistance.

T-TUBES, J-TUBES, AND PENROSE DRAINS

T-tubes are usually used for post-operative drainage of the common bile duct following common bile duct exploration or choledochotomy (Fig. 16–11). A T-tube cholangiogram is commonly performed on the seventh to tenth post-operative day; if the cholangiogram is normal, the T-tube is removed; if a blockage

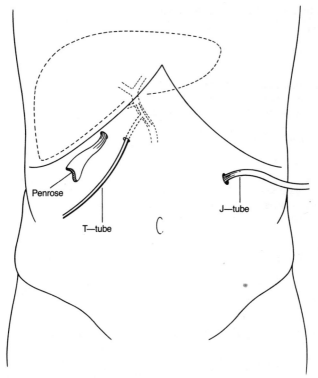

Figure 16–11. T-tube, J-tube, and Penrose drain.

(strictures, tumors, retained common duct stones) exists the T-tube is left in place.

J-tubes are jejunostomy tubes inserted to provide enteral nutrition on a long-term basis. *Gastrostomy tubes* may be inserted percutaneously under direct vision (e.g., gastroscopy or fluoroscopy).

Penrose drains are flat rubber drains inserted into wounds or operative sites with potential dead spaces, to prevent the accumulation of pus, intestinal contents, blood, bile, or pancreatic juice.

Closed suction (Davon or Jackson-Pratt) *drains* are used with operative, large potential dead spaces where bacterial ingress may contaminate sterile cavities.

Sump drains have filters incorporated into them to prevent airborne bacteria from entering; they are usually used to drain peripancreatic fluid collections. Interventional radiologists sometimes insert various percutaneous drains into the biliary tree and intra-abdominal abscesses. Problems with these drains should be referred to the radiologist or surgeon.

Blocked T-Tubes and J-Tubes

Phone Call

Questions

1. **How long has the tube been blocked?**
2. **What type of tube is in place?**
3. **Has the tube been dislodged?**
4. **What operation was performed and how many days ago?**
5. **What are the vital signs?**
6. **What was the reason for admission?**

Orders

Ask the RN for a dressing set, two pairs of gloves in your size, and chlorhexidine (Hibitane) skin disinfectant to be at the bedside. You will have to remove the dressing around the drainage tube, and you must keep the site sterile.

Inform RN

"Will arrive at the bedside in . . . minutes."

Provided you are certain the tube has not been dislodged, assessment of blocked T-tubes and J-tubes can wait an hour or two if other problems of higher priority exist.

Elevator Thoughts (What causes blocked T-tubes or J-tubes?)

1. Blood clots within the tube
2. Debris within the tube
3. Failure to irrigate the tube regularly

Major Threat to Life

■ Sepsis with blocked T-tubes

Blocked T-tubes may lead to post-operative infection with resultant abscess formation or systemic sepsis. Blocked J-tubes, provided they are not dislodged, present no immediate threat to life. The risk of further surgery exists, if replacement of the tube is required.

Bedside

Quick Look Test

Does the patient look well (comfortable), sick (uncomfortable or distressed), or critical (about to die)?

The patient with a blocked T-tube or J-tube will look well, unless the underlying problem causes the patient to look sick or critical.

Airway and Vital Signs

A blocked T-tube or J-tube should not compromise the airway or the vital signs.

Selective Physical Examination and Management

Aspirate and irrigate the tube as follows:

1. Ask an assistant to hold the distal part of the T-tube or J-tube close to the connection between the tube and the drainage bag.
2. Wear sterile gloves and clean the distal end of the T-tube or J-tube and the proximal connecting tubing with chlorhexidine (Hibitane).
3. Disconnect the tube from the connecting tubing and give the connecting tubing to the assistant to maintain a sterile field.
4. Using a 5-ml syringe, aspirate *very gently* (i.e., withdraw the syringe plunger) to dislodge and extract the obstruction.
5. If this maneuver is unsuccessful, fill a second 5-ml syringe with 3 ml of sterile NS and *very gently* flush the T-tube or J-tube by applying slow, careful pressure to the syringe plunger. Only gentle pressure should be used. After flushing with saline, attempt to aspirate gently. If this maneuver fails, *do not try again*.
6. Reconnect the T-tube or J-tube and the drainage bag, maintaining sterile technique.

If aspiration and irrigation are unsuccessful, the surgeon should be informed immediately. The decision between a T-tube cholangiogram to visualize the problem or a closed exploration of the obstructed tube with Fogarty's catheter will have to be made. Closed exploration should be performed only by someone experienced in the procedure; it can be done only when a large, intact T-tube has been used or when the back wall of the T-limb has been cut away. An adequately functioning T-tube usually drains 100 to 250 ml/8 hr.

Dislodged T-Tubes, J-Tubes, and Penrose Drains

Phone Call

Questions

1. **How long ago was the tube or drain dislodged?**
2. **What type of tube is in place?**
3. **What operation was performed and how many days ago?**
4. **What are the vital signs?**
5. **What was the reason for admission?**

Orders

Ask the RN for a dressing set, two pairs of gloves in your size, and chlorhexidine (Hibitane) skin cleanser to be at the bedside.

You will have to remove the dressing around the drainage tube, and you must keep the site sterile.

Inform RN

"Will arrive at the bedside in . . . minutes."

Assessment of dislodged T-tubes and J-tubes requires you to see the patient immediately, since urgent replacement of the tube is mandatory, if it was inserted recently. A delay in this replacement may result in the patient's requiring emergency surgery to replace the tube.

Elevator Thoughts (What causes dislodgement of tubes and drains?)

1. Failure to secure the tube or drain adequately
2. Confused, uncooperative patient

Major Threat to Life

■ Sepsis

Dislodged T-tubes and Penrose drains may lead to post-operative sepsis with resultant abscess formation or systemic sepsis. Dislodged J-tubes and T-tubes that cannot be replaced early may require surgical replacement, thus increasing the risk of morbidity and mortality from a second anesthetic.

Bedside

Quick Look Test

Does the patient look well (comfortable), sick (uncomfortable or distressed), or critical (about to die)?

The patient with a recently dislodged T-tube, J-tube, or Penrose drain will look well unless the underlying problem causes the patient to look sick or critical.

Airway and Vital Signs

A dislodged T-tube, J-tube, or Penrose drain should not compromise the vital signs acutely.

Selective Physical Examination and Management

A dislodged *T-tube* draining the common bile duct is a potentially life-threatening situation since septic shock can follow rapidly. If dislodgement is suspected order an immediate T-tube cholangiogram and inform the surgeon. The patient will need surgery to re-establish drainage, if the dislodgement is confirmed by the cholangiogram.

A dislodged *J-tube* (enterostomy tube) must be re-inserted immediately as follows:

1. Wear sterile gloves and clean and drape the tube exit site.
2. If the tube is only partially dislodged, carefully clean the exposed tubing and gently advance the tube to the appropriate (previous) depth.
3. If the tube has been completely dislodged, select a similar sterile tube and introduce it gently through the track left by the previous tube. *Do not force the tube.*
4. If this maneuver is successful, secure the tube well by suturing it in place with a 3–0 suture.
5. Order a water-soluble radiocontrast scan to confirm the correct positioning of the replaced or repositioned tube.

If replacement of the J-tube (enterostomy tube) is unsuccessful, notify the surgeon who will decide if an urgent re-operation is indicated.

Dislodged *Penrose drains* should not be reinserted into the wound since bacteria will be introduced into the site. Secure the Penrose drain in the position you find it and clinically examine the area for abscess formation (heat, tenderness, swelling) daily, for the next few days. Inform the surgeon that the Penrose drain has become dislodged.

NASOGASTRIC AND ENTERAL FEEDING TUBES

Blocked Nasogastric and Enteral Tubes

Phone Call

Questions

1. **How long has the tube been blocked?**
2. **What type of tube is in place?**
3. **Has the tube been dislodged?**
4. **What are the vital signs?**
5. **What was the reason for admission?**

Orders
Ask the RN for a 50-ml syringe, sterile NS, and a bowl to be at bedside.

Inform RN
"Will arrive at the bedside in . . . minutes."

A blocked NG or enteral tube is not an emergency. Assessment can wait an hour or two if other problems of a higher priority exist.

Elevator Thoughts (What causes blocked NG or enteral feeding tubes?)

- Debris within the tube
- Blood clots within the tube

■ Failure to irrigate the tube regularly

Major Threat to Life

■ Aspiration pneumonia

If the NG tube is blocked and thus fails to drain the stomach, gastric contents can be aspirated into the lungs.

Bedside

Quick Look Test
Does the patient look well (comfortable), sick (uncomfortable or distressed), or critical (about to die)?
Failure to drain the gastric contents by a blocked NG tube may result in the patient's developing nausea and vomiting, thus looking sick.

Airway and Vital Signs
What is the RR?
A blocked NG tube should not compromise the airway unless gastric contents accumulate and are aspirated into the lungs.

Selective Physical Examination and Management

1. Irrigate the tube with 25 to 50 ml of NS. As the tube is being irrigated, listen over the stomach region for the gurgling of fluid that indicates the tube is in the stomach.
2. If the previous maneuver is unsuccessful, remove the tube. If you are able to flush and clear the tube now, you may re-insert the same tube. However, if you are unsuccessful at flushing the tube, a new tube will be needed.
3. Ensure the usual nursing protocols are being followed for regular irrigation of the tube.

Dislodged Nasogastric and Enteral Feeding Tubes

Phone Call

Questions

1. **How long has the tube been dislodged?**
2. **What type of tube is in place?**
3. **What are the vital signs?**
4. **What was the reason for admission?**

Orders
Nil

Inform RN

"Will arrive at the bedside in . . . minutes."

Assessment of a dislodged NG or enteral feeding tube may wait an hour or two, if other problems of a higher priority exist. Be careful, however, not to leave the diabetic patient who has received insulin without caloric intake for too long.

Elevator Thoughts (What causes an NG or enteral feeding tube to become dislodged?)

- Failure to secure the tube adequately
- Confused, uncooperative patient

Major Threat to Life

- Aspiration pneumonia

If the NG tube is dislodged and thus fails to drain the stomach, gastric contents may accumulate and can be aspirated into the lung. The danger of a dislodged or misplaced enteral feeding tube is the risk of infusing the enteral feeding solution into the lung.

Bedside

Quick Look Test

Does the patient look well (comfortable), sick (uncomfortable or distressed), or critical (about to die)?

Patients who have aspirated because of a dislodged NG tube or a malpositioned feeding tube may appear tachypneic and unwell.

Airway and Vital Signs

A dislodged NG or enteral feeding tube should not compromise the vital signs, unless aspiration of gastric contents or enteral feeding solutions has occurred.

Selective Physical Examination and Management

1. Inspect the tube. **Are there any markings on the tube that indicate how far in the tube is situated?** If you are not familiar with these markings, ask the RN to bring a similar tube so you will be able to estimate how far in the tube is.
2. Aspirate the tube to see if gastric contents can be obtained. Instill 25 to 50 ml of air using the 50-ml syringe, while listening over the stomach region with your stethoscope. If the tube is properly positioned you should be able to hear a gurgling "swoosh," as air is introduced into the stomach.
3. A small bore enteral feeding tube should not be pushed farther down if it has been dislodged. Do *not* insert the guidewire down the tube blindly, as laceration or perforation of the esophagus,

stomach, or duodenum may occur if the tip of the guidewire exits from one of the distal apertures in the tube. Dislodged enteral feeding tubes must be removed and replaced. The same tube may be reused, with the guidewire being inserted into the tube under direct vision. The tube, stiffened by the guidewire, may then be reinserted.

4. Ensure the usual nursing protocols are being followed for regular irrigation of the tube.

17

POLYURIA-FREQUENCY-INCONTINENCE

You will receive many calls at night regarding patients' urinary volumes. Either the patients are voiding too much or too little. It is often difficult for a patient to differentiate between the problems of *polyuria* and *frequency* and, for many elderly patients, either one of these problems may present as *incontinence*. Once you clarify which one of the three problems is present, you will find the rest easy.

PHONE CALL

Questions

1. Clarify the symptom.
   Polyuria refers to a urine output of greater than 3 L/day. This usually comes to the attention of the nurse when reviewing the fluid balance record or when the urinary drainage bag needs frequent emptying. *Frequency* of urination refers to the frequent passage of urine, whether of large or small volume, and may occur in concert with polyuria or urinary incontinence.
   Urinary incontinence is a major problem in elderly patients and a frequent source of frustration for nurses. Avoid ordering Foley's catheter as the first line of treatment.
2. **What are the vital signs?**
3. **What was the admitting diagnosis?**

Orders

1. If the patient is hypotensive order a large bore IV (#16 if possible) immediately, if not already in place. (Refer to Chapter 15 for further investigation and management of hypotension.)
2. Urinalysis, urine culture. Urinary tract infections in this group of patients are sufficiently common to warrant these studies when called for any of these three problems.

Inform RN

"Will arrive at bedside in . . . minutes."
Polyuria, frequency, and incontinence are seldom urgent problems. However, the concomitant presence of hypotension will require you to see the patient immediately.

ELEVATOR THOUGHTS

What causes *polyuria?*

- Diabetes mellitus
- Diabetes insipidus (central; nephrogenic)
- Psychogenic polydipsia
- Large volumes of oral or IV fluids
- Diuretics
- Diuretic phase of acute tubular necrosis
- Salt losing nephritis

What causes *frequency?*

- Urinary tract infection
- Partial bladder outlet obstruction (e.g., prostatism)
- Bladder irritation (tumors, stones, infections)

What causes *incontinence?*

- Urinary tract infection
- Detrusor instability (stroke, Alzheimer's disease, normal pressure hydrocephalus, prostatic hypertrophy, pelvic tumor)
- Stress incontinence (in multiparous women, lax pelvic bladder support; in men, after prostatic surgery)
- Overflow incontinence (bladder outlet obstruction as in BPH, urethral stricture; spinal cord disease, autonomic neuropathy)
- Environmental factors (inaccessibility to call bell, "obstacle course" to the bathroom)
- Iatrogenic factors (diuretics, sedatives)

MAJOR THREAT TO LIFE

- *Polyuria*: Hypovolemic shock

If polyuria is not due to fluid excess, and continues without adequate fluid replacement, the intravascular volume will drop, and the patient will become hypotensive.

- *Frequency* or *incontinence*: Septic shock

Frequency or incontinence does not pose a major threat to life unless an underlying urinary tract infection goes unchecked and progresses to pyelonephritis or septic shock.

BEDSIDE

Quick Look Test

Does the patient look well (comfortable), sick (uncomfortable or distressed), or critical (about to die)?

It is unusual for the patient to look anything but well. If sick or critical, search for a separate unrecognized problem.

Airway and Vital Signs

Check for postural changes. A rise in HR >15 beats/min or a fall in systolic BP > 15 mm Hg or any fall in diastolic BP indicates significant hypovolemia. *Caution*: A resting tachycardia alone may indicate decreased intravascular volume.

Fever suggests possible urinary tract infection.

Selective Physical Examination I

Is the patient volume depleted?

CVS   Pulse volume, JVP
         Skin temperature and color
NEURO   Level of consciousness

Management

What immediate measure needs to be taken to correct or prevent hypovolemic shock?

Replace Intravascular Volume. If volume depleted, give IV NS or Ringer's lactate, aiming for a JVP of 2 to 3 cm H_2O above the sternal angle and normalization of the vital signs. Remember that aggressive fluid repletion in a patient with a history of CHF may compromise cardiac function. Do not overshoot the mark!

Selective History and Chart Review

Identify the specific problem.

Polyuria. The assessment of polyuria can be estimated by history but accurately confirmed only by scrutiny of meticulously kept fluid balance sheets. If these are not available order strict input/output monitoring. It is worthwhile to document polyuria (> 3 L/day) before embarking on an exhaustive workup of a non-existent problem.

1. Ask about associated symptoms. "Polyuria + polydipsia" suggests diabetes mellitus, diabetes insipidus, or compulsive water drinking (psychogenic polydipsia). Of these, diabetes mellitus is the most common.
2. Check the chart for recent laboratory results.
    a. Blood glucose (diabetes mellitus)
    b. Potassium
    c. Calcium
   Hypokalemia and hypercalcemia are important reversible causes of nephrogenic diabetes insipidus. Refer to Chapter 27 for management of hypokalemia; Chapter 24 for management of hypercalcemia.
3. Make sure the patient is not on any drugs that may cause either nephrogenic diabetes insipidus (lithium carbonate, demeclocycline) or diuresis (diuretics, aminophylline).

Frequency. Frequency can be assessed by questioning the patient; estimate from the nursing notes or fluid balance sheets if the patient is an unreliable historian. Ask about associated symptoms. Fever, dysuria, hematuria, and foul smelling urine suggest urinary tract infection. Poor stream, hesitancy, dribbling, or nocturia suggests prostatism.

Incontinence. Incontinence is obvious when it occurs and is often embarrassing to the patient. You need an honest history from the patient in order to make a proper diagnosis. Address the subject non-judgmentally.

Selective Physical Examination II

Look for specific causes and complications of polyuria, frequency, or incontinence.

VITALS	Fever (UTI)
HEENT	Visual fields (pituitary neoplasm)
	Acetone breath (diabetic ketoacidosis)
RESP	Kussmaul's respirations (diabetic ketoacidosis)
	Kussmaul's respirations are characterized by deep, pauseless breathing at a rate of 25 to 30/min.
ABD	Enlarged bladder (neurogenic bladder)
	Suprapubic tenderness (cystitis)
NEURO	Level of consciousness
	Localizing findings
	An alert, conscious person with polyuria and with free access to fluids and salt will not become volume depleted. If volume depletion is present, suspect metabolic or structural neurologic abnormalities impairing the normal response to thirst. Perform a complete neurologic examination, looking for evidence of stroke, subdural hemorrhage, or metabolic abnormalities.
SKIN	Perineal skin breakdown (a complication of repeated incontinence and a source of infection)
RECTAL	Enlarged prostate (bladder outlet obstruction)
	Perineal sensation, resting tone of anal sphincter, anal wink, bulbocavernosus reflex.
	An anal wink is elicited by gently stroking the perianal mucosa with a tongue depressor. A normal response is manifested by contraction of the external anal sphincter.
	To elicit the bulbocavernosus reflex, the index finger of the examining hand is introduced into the rectum, and the patient is asked to relax the sphincter as much as possible. The glans penis is then squeezed

with the opposite hand, which normally results in involuntary contraction of the anal sphincter.

Innervation of the anus is similar to that of the lower urinary tract. Therefore, abnormalities in perineal sensation or in the sacral reflexes may provide the clue that a spinal cord lesion is responsible for the incontinence.

Management

What more needs to be done tonight?

Polyuria

1. Once intravascular volume is restored, ensure adequate continuing replacement (usually IV) fluid as estimated by urinary, insensible (400 to 800 ml/day), and other (nasogastric suction, vomiting, diarrhea) losses. Re-check the volume status periodically to ensure that your mathematic estimates for replacement correlate with an appropriate clinical response.
2. Order strict intake/output records to be kept.
3. Serum glucose, Chemstrip, or Glucometer testing. This will identify diabetes mellitus before it progresses to ketoacidosis (IDDM) or hyperosmolar coma (NIDDM). The presence of glycosuria on urinalysis will provide more rapid evidence of hyperglycemia as a possible cause of polyuria.

   Random blood glucose levels of < 10 mmol/L are seldom accompanied by osmotic diuresis. If hyperglycemia of more than 10 mmol/L exists refer to Chapter 26, page 259, for further management.
4. Serum calcium level is often not available as a stat test at night. If there is strong suspicion of hypercalcemia (polyuria or lethargy in a patient with malignancy, hyperparathyroidism, or sarcoidosis) contact the laboratory for permission to measure serum calcium level on an urgent basis.
5. Maximal urine concentrating ability measured by the water deprivation test can help differentiate among central diabetes insipidus, nephrogenic diabetes insipidus, and psychogenic polydipsia. This test can be arranged on an elective basis in the morning.

Frequency

1. If other symptoms (urgency, dysuria, low grade fever, suprapubic tenderness) of urinary tract infection (cystitis) are present empiric teatment with antibiotics is warranted, pending urine culture and sensitivity results which will usually take 48 hours to complete. *Amoxicillin* 500 mg PO q8h for 7 to 10 days or *trimethoprim-sulfamethoxazole* (Septra D.S.) (160 mg–800 mg), 1 tablet PO BID for 7 to 10 days may be used.

   In young outpatient females, single dose therapy has been

successful, e.g., *amoxicillin* 3 gm PO × 1 dose or *trimethoprim-sulfamethoxazole* (160 mg–800 mg) PO × 1 dose. However, these single dose regimens have not been definitely proved efficacious in the hospitalized population.

Allergies to penicillin and its derivatives and to sulfonamides are common. Ensure absence of allergies to these drugs before initiating treatment. If allergic to penicillin and to sulfonamides, *cephalexin* (Keflex) 500 mg PO QID for 7 days can be given, recognizing a 10 to 15% cross-reactivity in penicillin-allergic patients. Inform these patients of this risk.

Phenazopyridine (Pyridium) 200 mg PO TID after meals may help alleviate dysuria in cases of urethritis during the first day or two of treatment. Warn the patient that this drug may turn the urine orange. Also, encourage high fluid intake to promote "washout" of the urinary tract.

2. If history and physical examination suggest partial bladder outlet obstruction examine the abdomen carefully for an enlarged bladder. If in urinary retention a Foley's catheter should be placed. (Refer to Chapter 7, page 57, for further investigation and management of urinary retention.)

Always check for heart murmurs before catheterizing a patient. A patient with a cardiac valvular abnormality is at risk for development of infectious endocarditis following GU procedures, including catheterization with a Foley's catheter. Any patient with a documented valvular abnormality, including mitral valve prolapse with a persistent systolic murmur, should receive antibiotic prophylaxis directed primarily against enterococci prior to catheterization. Current recommendations are as follows: *ampicillin,* 2 gm IM or IV, plus *gentamicin,* 1.5 mg/kg IM or IV. Both antibiotics should be given 30 minutes prior to the procedure and once again 8 hours later.

Patients who are allergic to penicillin may be treated with *vancomycin* 1 gm IV over 1 hr, plus *gentamicin* 1.5 mg/kg IM or IV. Both of these antibiotics should be given 1 hour prior to the procedure and once again 8 to 12 hours later.

3. Other causes of frequency, such as bladder irritation by stones or tumor, can be addressed by urologic consultation in the morning. You may be able to expedite the diagnosis of bladder tumor by ordering a collection of urine for cytology.

Incontinence

1. Even if incontinence is the only symptom, order a urinalysis and urine culture to ensure that a urinary tract infection is not contributing to the patient's symptoms.
2. Check for hyperglycemia, hypokalemia, and hypercalcemia if there is a question of polyuria. These conditions may present as incontinence in the elderly or bedridden patient, and their proper treatment may alleviate the incontinence.

3. If neurologic examination (e.g., abnormal sacral reflexes, diminished perineal sensation, lower limb weakness or spasticity) suggests the presence of a *spinal cord lesion* consultation should be arranged with a neurologist.

4. In the case of *overflow incontinence,* intermittent straight catheterization q4 to 6h is preferable to an indwelling Foley's catheter, as it is less likely to cause infection. Aim for a urine volume of less than 400 ml q4 to 6h. Greater volumes result in ureterovesical reflux, which promotes ascending urinary tract infection. A young motivated patient with a neurogenic bladder can be taught to self-catheterize.

   Though not ideal, long-term indwelling Foley's catheters are occasionally necessary when insufficient nursing services preclude frequent intermittent catheterizations. In these cases, a silicone elastomer (Silastic) Foley catheter should be used. This type has the advantage of less predisposition to calcification and encrustation and may be kept in place up to 6 weeks at a time.

5. *Detrusor instability* is a condition in which the bladder escapes central inhibition, resulting in reflex contractions. It is the most common cause of incontinence in the elderly population and is often manifested by *urge incontinence* (involuntary micturition preceded by a warning of a few seconds or minutes). Ensure that there are no physical barriers preventing the patient from reaching the bathroom or commode in time.

   Is there easy access to the call bell? Are the nurses responding promptly? Are the bedrails kept up or down? Does the patient have a medical condition (e.g., Parkinson's disease, stroke, arthritis) that prevents easy mobilization when the urge to void occurs?

   If there is no evidence of perineal skin breakdown, *urinary incontinence pads* with frequent checks and changes by the nursing staff are entirely adequate. (Babies exist for years in such a state!) If perineal skin breakdown or ulceration is present, a Foley's or condom catheter is justified to allow skin healing.

6. Urinary spillage with coughing or straining suggests *stress incontinence.* Again, if there is no evidence of perineal skin breakdown, urinary incontinence pads are perfectly adequate until urologic consultation can assess the need for surgery.

Remember

Urinary incontinence is an understandable source of frustration for nurses' caring for these patients. Listen to the concerns of the nurses' looking after your patients and discuss with them the reasons for your actions.

18

PRONOUNCING DEATH

One of the required duties of medical students and interns on-call at night is the pronouncement of death in patients who have recently expired. This is a situation that is seldom addressed in medical school, and you will certainly wonder what needs to be done in order to pronounce a patient dead. Unfortunately, there has long been uncertainty surrounding what constitutes the medical and legal definition of death.

Traditionally, the determination of death has been solely a medical decision. In the United States, legislative action on the criteria of death falls within state jurisdiction. Many states have opted to follow the recommendations set forth by the Harvard Medical School Ad Hoc Committee,[1] Capron and Kass,[2] or the Kansas legislation of 1971.[3] It is best to be familiar with the medical and legal criteria accepted for the determination of death in the particular state in which you work.

The recommended criteria of death to be used for all purposes within the jurisdiction of the Parliament of Canada, issued by the Law Reform Commission of Canada[4] in 1981 were as follows:

1. A person is dead when an irreversible cessation of all that person's brain function has occurred.
2. The irreversible cessation of brain function can be determined by the prolonged absence of spontaneous circulatory and respiratory functions.
3. When the determination of the prolonged absence of spontaneous circulatory and respiratory functions is made impossible by the use of artificial means of support, the irreversible cessation of the brain function can be determined by any means recognized by the ordinary standards of current medical practice.

Although criterion 1 alone may imply that a complete neurologic examination is required for pronouncement of death, we know that this is neither practical nor necessary. Criterion 2 accounts for this by assuming that when "prolonged absence of spontaneous circulatory and respiratory functions" exists, irreversible cessation of the patient's brain function has occurred. Hence, there will be no question in the majority of cases that most of the patients you will be asked to pronounce dead will indeed be medically and legally dead, as they will fulfill the criterion set out in 2 alone. Thus, legally, in most cases all that is required of you to pronounce a patient dead is to verify that there has been a prolonged absence of spontaneous circulatory and respiratory functions. A slightly more detailed assessment is recommended, however, and will take only a few minutes to complete.

The RN will page you and inform you of the death of the patient, requesting that you come to the unit and pronounce the patient dead.

1. Identify the patient by the hospital identification tag worn on the wrist.
2. Ascertain that the patient does not rouse to verbal or tactile stimuli.
3. Listen for heart sounds and feel for the carotid pulse. The deceased patient is pulseless and without heart sounds.
4. Look and listen to the patient's chest for evidence of spontaneous respirations. The deceased patient shows no evidence of breathing movements or of air entry on examination.
5. Record the position of the pupils and their reaction to light. The deceased patient shows no evidence of pupillary reaction to light. Though the pupils are usually dilated, this position is not invariable.
6. Record the time at which your assessment was completed. Although other emergencies take precedence over pronouncing a patient dead, one should try not to postpone this task too long, as the time of death is legally the time at which you pronounce the patient dead.
7. Document your findings on the chart. A typical chart entry may read as follows: Called to pronounce Mr. Doe dead. Patient unresponsive to verbal or tactile stimuli. No heart sounds heard, no pulse felt. Not breathing, no air entry heard. Pupils fixed and dilated. Patient pronounced dead at 2030 hours, December 7, 1987.
8. Notify the family physician, attending physician, or both if the nurses have not already done so. Decide together with the attending physician whether an autopsy would be useful and appropriate in this patient's case.
9. Notification of relatives. Next of kin should be notified as soon as possible after you have pronounced the patient dead and notified the family physician, attending physician, or both. Normally, it is the responsibility of the family physician to notify the relatives once he has been told of the patient's death.

   Occasionally, you may experience the situation where the family physician has signed over his or her night-time call to a partner or another physician who does not know the patient or family. In this situation it is best to inform the physician on-call and, if he or she is uncomfortable with speaking to the family, a member of the house staff who knows the patient or family best should then notify the next of kin. The family will appreciate hearing the news from a familiar voice.

   If neither the family physician on call nor the house staff knows the patient, spend a few minutes familiarizing yourself with the patient's medical history and mode of death. If you are appointed to deliver the news to the family, the following guidelines may be helpful.

a. Identify yourself; e.g., "This is Dr. Jones calling from St. Paul's Hospital."

b. Ask for the next of kin; e.g., "May I speak to Mrs. Doe, please?"

c. Deliver the message; e.g., "Mrs. Doe, I am sorry to inform you that your husband died at 8:30 this evening."

d. You may be surprised to find that in many instances this news is not unexpected. It is, however, always comforting to a family to know that a relative has died peacefully; e.g., "As you know your husband was suffering from a terminal illness. Although I was not with your husband at the time of his death, the nurses looking after him assure me that he was very comfortable at the time of his death and that he passed away peacefully."

e. If an autopsy is desired by one of the medical staff, this question should be broached now; e.g., "Your husband had an unusual illness, and if you are agreeable, it would be very useful to us to perform an autopsy. Although it obviously won't change the course of events in terms of your husband's illness, it may provide some valuable information for other patient's suffering from similar problems to your husband's." If there is any hesitation on the part of the next of kin, emphasize that they are under no obligation to grant permission for an autopsy to be performed if it is against the perceived wishes of the patient or family.

   If the next of kin refuses, do not argue, no matter how interested you may be in the outcome of the case. Accept the family's decision graciously; e.g., "We understand completely and, of course, we will respect your wishes."

f. Ask the next of kin if he or she would like to come to the hospital to see the patient one last time. Inform the nurses of this decision. Questions pertaining to funeral homes and the patient's personal belongings are best referred to the nurse in charge.

SPECIAL SITUATIONS

Medical technology has introduced two other scenarios in the pronouncement of a patient's death.

The Mechanically Ventilated Patient without Circulatory Function. There is general understanding that those patients whose hearts have stopped beating despite being mechanically ventilated will all meet the criteria for legal death, through a lack of spontaneous ventilation once the ventilator is turned off. Thus, it is reasonable practice to

1. Ensure that connections are intact and properly attached if the patient is on the ECG monitor. (This assures that the absence of cardiac electrical activity is not an artifact due to faulty electrical connections.)
2. Follow the usual procedure for pronouncing death.
3. Discuss your findings with the attending physician *before* disconnecting the ventilator.
4. After agreement with the attending physician, disconnect the ventilator. Observe the patient for 3 minutes for evidence of spontaneous respiration.
5. Document your findings in the chart; e.g., called to pronounce Mr. Doe dead. Patient unresponsive to verbal or tactile stimuli. No heart sounds heard; no pulse felt. Pupils fixed and dilated. Patient being mechanically ventilated. Ventilator disconnected at 2030 hours after discussion with attending physician, Dr. Smith. No spontaneous respirations noted for 3 minutes. Patient pronounced dead at 2033 hours, December 7, 1987.

The Mechanically Ventilated Patient with Circulatory Function Intact. This type of patient is usually being cared for in the ICU. A variety of controversial criteria exists for the determination of brain death, and criteria may differ between geographic locations. The task of pronouncing a mechanically ventilated patient dead and the discussion of organ procurement are best left to the ICU staff and associated subspecialists in consultation with the patient's family.

REFERENCES

1. Report of the Ad Hoc Committee of the Harvard Medical School to Examine the Definition of Brain Death. J.A.M.A. 205, 337 (1968).
2. Capron and Kass. A Statutory Definition of the Standards for Determining Human Death, 121 U. PA. L. Rev. 87 (1972a).
3. Kan. Stat. Ann. 77–202 (Supp. 1974).
4. Report on the Criteria for the Determination of Death. Law Reform Commission of Canada, 1981.

19

SEIZURES

A seizure is one of the more dramatic events you may witness while on-call. Usually everyone around you will be in a panic. The key to controlling the situation is to remain calm.

PHONE CALL

Questions

1. **Is the patient still seizing?**
2. **What type of seizure was witnessed? Was the seizure grand mal (generalized tonic-clonic) or was it focal?**
3. **What is the patient's level of consciousness?**
4. **Has there been any obvious injury?**
5. **What was the reason for admission?**
6. **Does the patient have diabetes mellitus?**

Orders

1. Ask the RN to make sure the patient is positioned on his or her side. During both the seizure and the postictal state the patient should be kept in the lateral decubitus position to prevent aspiration of gastric contents.
2. Ask the RN to have the following available *at the bedside*:
   a. Oral airway
   b. IV set-up with NS (flushed through and ready for immediate use)
   c. Two blood tubes (one for chemistry and one for hematology)
   d. *Diazepam* (Valium) 20 mg
   e. *Thiamine* 100 mg
   f. D50W 50 ml (1 ampule)
   g. Chart
3. If the patient is postictal, ask the RN to remove any dentures, suction the oropharynx, and insert an oral airway.
4. Order a stat blood glucose, Chemstrip, or Glucometer reading if the patient is in the postictal state (unconscious).

Inform RN

"Will arrive at bedside in . . . minutes."
A seizure requires you to see the patient immediately.

ELEVATOR THOUGHTS (What causes seizures?)

Drugs

1. Anti-epileptic medication inadvertently discontinued or non-therapeutic level
2. Alcohol withdrawal. *Caution*: **Does the patient have delirium tremens in addition to the seizures?**
3. Meperidine (Demerol) overdose (an easily missed diagnosis in the elderly post-operative patient)
4. Benzodiazepine withdrawal
5. Penicillin at high doses
6. Theophylline toxicity

CNS

1. Tumor
2. Previous stroke
3. Previous head injury
4. Meningitis/encephalitis
5. Idiopathic epilepsy

ENDO

1. Hypoglycemia
2. Hyponatremia ⎫
3. Hypocalcemia ⎬ "The four hypos"
4. Hypomagnesemia ⎭

MISC

1. Uremia
2. CNS vasculitis
3. Hypertensive encephalopathy
4. Hypoxia/hypercapnia
5. Pseudoseizure

MAJOR THREAT TO LIFE

- Aspiration
- Hypoxia

The patient should be lying in the left lateral decubitus position to prevent the tongue from falling posteriorly, blocking the airway, and to minimize the risk of aspiration of gastric contents while in the postictal state. Patients usually keep breathing throughout seizure activity. Most patients can be in status epilepticus for 90 minutes with no subsequent neurologic damage.

The majority of seizures will have stopped by the time you arrive at the bedside. The procedures and protocols to follow if the seizure has stopped are discussed subsequently. The procedures and protocols to follow if the seizure persists begin on page 194.

SEIZURE HAS STOPPED

Bedside

Quick Look Test

Does the patient look well (comfortable), sick (uncomfortable or distressed), or critical (about to die)?

Most patients after a grand mal seizure are unconscious (the postictal state).

Airway, Vital Signs, and Blood Glucose Results

In what position is the patient lying?

The patient should be positioned in the lateral decubitus position to prevent aspiration of gastric contents (Fig. 19–1).

Remove any dentures and suction the airway. Insert an oral airway if one is not already in place (Fig. 19–2). You are not out of the woods yet! The patient might begin to experience another seizure, so make sure the airway is protected.

Give oxygen by face mask or nasal prongs.

What is the Chemstrip result?

Hypoglycemia needs to be treated immediately to prevent further seizures.

Management I

Draw blood (20 ml) and establish IV access. Send the blood for the following tests:

Chemistry Tube

Electrolytes, urea, creatinine, random blood glucose, Ca, Mg, albumin, and antiepileptic drug levels, if the patient is receiving these medications. If the patient is undergoing a 3-day fast for investigation of possible hypoglycemia, order an insulin level as well.

Hematology Tube

CBC and manual differential.

Once the IV is established keep the line open with NS. NS is the IV fluid of choice. Phenytoin is not compatible with dextrose-containing solutions.

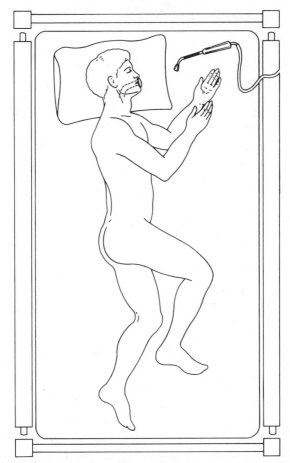

Figure 19–1. Positioning of the patient to prevent aspiration of gastric contents.

If the Chemstrip result or Glucometer reading reveals hypoglycemia give *thiamine* 100 mg IV by slow, direct injection over 3 to 5 minutes, followed by D50W 50 ml IV by slow, direct injection. Thiamine is given prior to the administration of glucose to protect against an exacerbation of Wernicke's encephalopathy.

Draw ABGs if the patient appears cyanotic.

Selective Physical Examination I

Assess LOC. **Does the patient respond to verbal or painful stimuli? Is the patient in a postictal state (i.e., decreased level of**

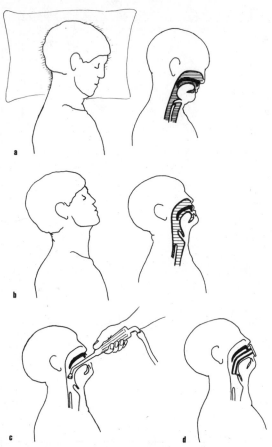

Figure 19–2. Airway management. Correct positioning of the head, correct suctioning, and correct inserting of an oral airway. a = neck flexion closes the airway, b = neck extension to sniffing position opens the airway, c = suctioning, and d = placement of the airway.

consciousness)? Remember, if the patient does not regain consciousness between seizures, after 30 minutes the diagnosis becomes *status epilepticus.*

Selective History and Chart Review

Ask any witnesses the following details about the seizure:

- **Length of time?**
- **Grand mal or focal?**

- **Onset grand mal or focal?** A focal onset of a grand mal seizure suggests structural brain disease, which may be old or new.
- **Any injury observed during seizure?**

Is there a history of seizures, alcohol withdrawal, head injury (e.g., recent fall while in the hospital), stroke, CNS tumor (primary or secondary), or diabetes mellitus?
Is the patient receiving any of the following medications?

- Penicillin
- Meperidine (Demerol)
- Insulin
- Oral hypoglycemics
- Chlorpromazine (lowers the seizure threshold)
- Anti-epileptic drugs

What are the most recent laboratory results?

- Glucose
- Na
- Ca
- Albumin
- Mg
- Anti-epileptic drug levels
- Urea
- Creatinine

The chart is reviewed before the physical examination because an immediate, treatable cause (e.g., insulin or meperidine (Demerol) overdose, hyponatremia) is more likely to be found in the chart.

Selective Physical Examination II

VITALS	Repeat now.
HEENT	Tongue or cheek lacerations, nuchal rigidity
RESP	Signs of aspiration
NEURO	Complete CNS examination within the limits of LOC.
	Can the patient speak, follow commands?
	Is there any asymmetry of pupils, visual fields, reflexes, or plantar responses? Asymmetry suggests structural brain disease.
MSS	Palpate skull and face, spine and ribs
	Passive ROM of all four limbs
	Are there lacerations, hematomas, or fractures?

Management II

Establish the *provisional* and *differential diagnoses* of the seizure—this must be a *causally defined* diagnosis (e.g., "Grand mal seizure secondary to hypoglycemia").

Table 19–1. SEIZURE PRECAUTIONS

1. Bed placed in lowest position.
2. Oral airway at head of bed.
3. Side rails up when patient in bed. In case of grand mal seizure, the side rails should be padded.
4. Provide patient with a firm pillow.
5. Suction at bedside.
6. Oxygen at bedside.
7. Bathroom privileges with supervision only.
8. Baths or showers only with a nurse in attendance.
9. Axilla temperature only.
10. Smoking only under supervision.
11. Direct supervision when using sharp objects, e.g., straight razor, nail scissors.

Are there any *complications* **of the seizure giving rise to a second diagnosis?** For example, if a head injury has been sustained, the *provisional diagnosis* might be "forehead hematoma" and the *differential diagnosis* would include subdural hematoma, frontal bone fracture.

Treat the underlying cause! "Seizure" is a symptom not a diagnosis.

Maintain *IV access* for 24 hours with NS. If there is concern regarding volume overloading, use a heparin lock instead of maintaining the IV open with NS.

It is not necessary to administer anti-epileptic medications unless there are inadequate serum concentrations or further seizures are anticipated (e.g., structural CNS abnormality, idiopathic epilepsy). If further seizures are anticipated, a long-acting anti-epileptic drug (e.g., phenytoin rather than diazepam) is recommended (see page 197 for dosage). Although diazepam is useful as an anticonvulsant to halt seizures, it is not useful as a prophylactic. The anti-epileptic medication of choice is phenytoin.

Seizure precautions should be instituted for the next 48 hours and then reviewed (Table 19–1).

PATIENT IS STILL SEIZING

Don't panic (almost everybody else will)! Most seizures will resolve without treatment within 2 minutes.

Bedside

Quick Look Test

Does the patient look well (comfortable), sick (uncomfortable or distressed), or critical (about to die)?

A patient having a grand mal seizure often engenders anxiety in the observer. Remember, if the patient is seizing, you can be assured that he or she has both a BP and a pulse.

Ask the RN to notify your resident of the situation—a seizure is a medical emergency.

Airway, Vital Signs, and Blood Glucose Result

In what position is the patient lying?

The patient should be positioned and maintained in the lateral decubitus position, to prevent aspiration of gastric contents. One or two assistants may be required to hold the patient in this position, if the seizure is violent.

Suction the airway. Do *not* insert an oral airway or attempt to remove dentures if force is required; you will break the patient's teeth.

Give oxygen by face mask or nasal prongs.

What is the patient's BP?

It is virtually impossible to take a BP during a grand mal seizure, so palpate the femoral pulse. (You may need an assistant to hold the patient's knee against the bed.) A palpable femoral pulse indicates a systolic BP of >60 mm Hg.

What is the Chemstrip result?

Hypoglycemia needs to be treated immediately.

Management I

How long has the patient been seizing?

If the seizure has stopped refer to page 190.

If the Seizure Has Lasted < 3 Minutes

Do not give diazepam yet.

- Re-check the airway.
- Observe the seizure activity.
- Do *not* attempt to start an IV yet; it will be much easier in 1 or 2 minutes, after the seizure has stopped.
- Ensure IV tubing is flushed through with NS and that thiamine, D50W, diazepam, and two blood tubes are all available at the bedside.

If the Seizure Has Lasted > 3 Minutes

Draw blood (20 ml) and establish IV access.

Tips on Starting the IV

When the patient is seizing, it is very difficult to start an IV. This is an emergency and not the time for a novice to try their hand at starting an IV. Appoint the most experienced person present to obtain IV access. The patient's arm should be firmly held by one or two assistants (Fig. 19–3), while maintaining the

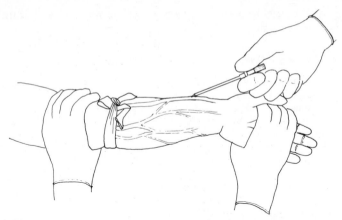

Figure 19–3. Positioning required when starting an IV during a grand mal seizure.

patient on the side. Sit down; it is much easier to start an IV when sitting rather than standing. Try for the largest blood vessel available but not the antecubital vein unless forced—since the elbow will then have to be splinted to avoid losing the IV access.

Medications

Order the following medications to be given immediately:

- *Thiamine* 100 mg IV by slow, direct injection over 3 to 5 minutes.
- D50W 50 ml IV by slow, direct injection. If hypoglycemic, the patient will become conscious abruptly while receiving the first 30 ml of D50W. Do not proceed with any further medication; change the IV to D5W. Thiamine is given prior to the administration of glucose to protect against an exacerbation of Wernicke's encephalopathy.

Diazepam

Give *diazepam* (Valium) at a rate of 2 mg/min IV, until the seizure stops or to a maximum dose of 20 mg. It will take 10 minutes to deliver 20 mg of diazepam at this rate. (An Ambu bag should be available at the bedside whenever diazepam is being given IV, since diazepam may cause respiratory depression.)

ABG

Draw ABGs.

Phenytoin

Ask an assistant to obtain the following:

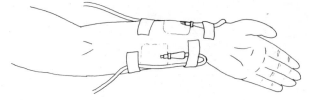

Figure 19–4. Two IVs are needed if both diazepam (Valium) and phenytoin (Dilantin) are to be administered.

- A second IV set-up with NS (Fig. 19–4).
- Phenytoin, loading dose 18 mg/kg (1250 mg for a 70 kg patient), to be available at the bedside.

The phenytoin loading dose may be injected directly via an NS IV at a rate no faster than 25 to 50 mg/min or as an *infusion,* (add the loading dose to 100 ml of NS) given at a rate not greater than 25 to 50 mg/min.

Second IV
Place a second IV (#16 if possible).
Diazepam and phenytoin are *not compatible,* so they cannot be given via the same IV.
Phenytoin may cause hypotension and cardiac dysrhythmias. Monitor the femoral pulse for decrease of volume (hypotension) and for irregularities of rhythm (Fig. 19–5). If either of these problems occurs, slow the phenytoin infusion rate.

Seizing Continues
If the patient is *still seizing* despite administering half the maximum dose of diazepam (10 mg), begin administering the loading dose of phenytoin (Dilantin) (no faster than 25 to 50 mg/min) but continue with the diazepam until the maximum dose has been given.
If the patient has *already received phenytoin* or has an inadequate level, give *half* the phenytoin loading dose IV. The most frequent side effects of "overshooting" with an extra loading dose are dizziness, nausea, and blurred vision for a few days. These are not major risks.

If the Seizure Now Stops
Stop giving the diazepam but give the full loading dose of phenytoin. Proceed to page 190 for further instructions. Most seizures can be controlled with diazepam and phenytoin—if not, CNS infection or structural brain disease should be considered.

If the Seizure Has Persisted for 30 Minutes
The patient is now in *status epilepticus*. This is an emergency! A

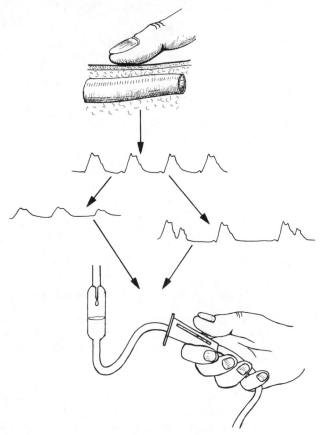

Figure 19–5. Phenytoin (Dilantin) may cause hypotension or cardiac dysrhythmias, detectable by palpating the femoral pulse. If either one is present, the phenytoin infusion rate should be slowed.

neurologist, intensivist, or anesthesiologist should be consulted immediately. The patient should be transferred to the ICU/CCU for management of the airway and probable intubation.

Status epilepticus is rare. It is defined as a single seizure lasting 30 minutes or repetitive seizures without intervening periods of normal consciousness, lasting more than 30 minutes.

While waiting for the ICU/CCU transfer and the neurology/ICU/anesthetic consultation proceed as follows:

1. *Phenobarbital* 8 to 20 mg/kg IV at a rate of 30 to 60 mg/min until the seizure stops.

OR

2. *Diazepam* infusion of 100 mg in 500 ml D5W to run at 40 ml/
hr. (Concentration = 8 mg/ml.)

If the Seizure Has Persisted for 60 Minutes
General anesthesia with halothane and neuromuscular blockade
is required.

REMEMBER

Seizures associated with head trauma or neurosurgery should be
treated with phenytoin alone, since other medications may depress
the level of consciousness.

20

Calls at night to assess a patient's breathing are common. Do not become overwhelmed by the myriad causes of SOB that you learned about in medical school. In hospitalized patients, as you will see, there are only four common causes of SOB.

PHONE CALL

Questions

1. **How long has the patient been SOB?**
2. **Did the SOB begin gradually or suddenly?**
   Sudden onset of SOB suggests pulmonary embolus or pneumothorax.
3. **Is the patient cyanosed?**
4. **What are the vital signs?**
5. **What was the reason for admission?**
6. **Does the patient have COPD?**
   What you really need to know is whether or not the patient is a CO_2 retainer. In most cases, this will apply to patients with COPD or with heavy smoking histories.
7. **Does the patient have O_2 ordered?**

Orders

1. Oxygen. If you are certain that the patient is not a CO_2 retainer you may safely order any concentration of O_2 in the short-term situation. If you are not certain order O_2 28% by Venturi's mask and reassess upon arrival at the bedside.
2. If the admitting diagnosis is *asthma* and the patient has not received a nebulized bronchodilator within the last 2 hours, order nebulized *salbutamol* (Ventolin) 2.5 to 5 mg in 3 ml NS immediately.
3. ABG set at bedside. Not all patients with SOB will require ABG determination, but it is best to have the equipment ready upon arrival if needed.

Inform RN

"Will arrive at bedside in . . . minutes."
SOB requires you to see the patient immediately.

ELEVATOR THOUGHTS (What causes SOB?)

Cardiovascular Causes

- CHF
- Pulmonary embolism

Pulmonary Causes

- Pneumonia
- Asthma/COPD (bronchospasm)

Miscellaneous Causes

- Anxiety, upper airway obstruction, pneumothorax, massive pleural effusions, massive ascites, post-operative atelectasis, pericardial tamponade

MAJOR THREAT TO LIFE

- Hypoxia

Inadequate tissue oxygenation is the most worrisome end result of any process causing SOB. Hence, you must direct your initial assessment towards ascertaining whether or not hypoxia is present.

BEDSIDE

Quick Look Test

Does the patient look well (comfortable), sick (uncomfortable or distressed), or critical (about to die)?
This simple observation will help determine the necessity of immediate intervention. If the patient looks sick, order ABGs, O_2, IV D5W TKVO, and a portable CXR immediately. If critical, begin manual ventilation with bag and mask, order IV D5W TKVO; ask the nurse to bring the cardiac arrest cart to the bedside, attach the patient to the ECG monitor, and prepare for possible intubation. Consult ICU immediately.

Airway and Vital Signs

Check that the upper airway is clear.

What is the respiratory rate?
Rates < 12/min suggest a central depression of ventilation, which is usually due to a stroke, narcotic overdose, or some other drug overdose. Rates > 20/min suggest hypoxia, pain, or anxiety. Look

also for thoracoabdominal dissociation that may indicate impending respiratory failure. Remember that the chest cage and abdominal wall normally move in the same direction.

What is the heart rate?
Sinus tachycardia is an expected accompaniment of hypoxia.

What is the temperature?
An elevated temperature suggests *infection* (pneumonia, pyothorax, or bronchitis) but is consistent with *pulmonary embolism.*

What is the BP?
Hypotension may indicate CHF, septic shock, massive pulmonary embolism, or tension pneumothorax (see Chapter 15). Also, measure the amount of *pulsus paradoxus* which, in asthmatics, roughly correlates with the degree of airflow obstruction. Pulsus paradoxus is an inspiratory fall in systolic BP > 10 mm Hg. To determine whether a pulsus paradoxus is present, inflate the BP cuff 20 to 30 mm Hg above the palpable systolic BP. Deflate the cuff slowly. Initially, Korotkoff's sounds will be heard only in expiration. At some point during cuff deflation Korotkoff's sounds will appear in inspiration as well, giving an impression of a doubling of the HR. The number of millimeters of mercury (mm Hg) between the initial appearance of Korotkoff's sounds and their appearance in inspiration represents the degree of pulsus paradoxus (Fig. 20–1).

Selective Physical Examination

Is the patient hypoxic?

VITALS   Repeat now. Again, ensure airway patency.
HEENT   Check for central cyanosis (blue tongue and mucous
                membranes).
                Check that the trachea is midline.
                Palpate for SC air in the neck or chest (pneumothorax).
RESP   Are breath sounds present and of normal intensity?
                Check for crackles, wheezing, consolidation, or
                pleural effusion.
NEURO   Check level of sensorium. Is the patient alert, confused,
                drowsy, or unresponsive?

Cyanosis often does not occur until there is severe hemoglobin desaturation and may not occur at all in the anemic patient. If hypoxia is suspected confirm by ABG measurement.

Management

What immediate measure needs to be taken to correct hypoxia?
Supply adequate O_2. The initial concentration of O_2 ordered

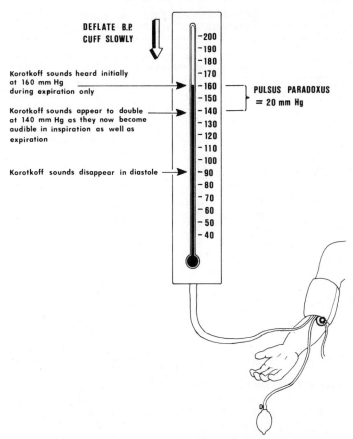

DEFLATE B.P. CUFF SLOWLY

Korotkoff sounds heard initially at 160 mm Hg during expiration only

Korotkoff sounds appear to double at 140 mm Hg as they now become audible in inspiration as well as expiration

Korotkoff sounds disappear in diastole

PULSUS PARADOXUS = 20 mm Hg

Figure 20–1. Determination of pulsus paradoxus.

depends on your judgment of how sick the patient is. An accurate assessment can be made by drawing ABG samples, beginning empiric O_2 treatment, and adjusting FIO_2, depending on the results of subsequent ABGs. Allow 20 to 30 minutes between ABG determinations. In most cases a $PO_2 > 60$ mm Hg or an O_2 saturation of 90% is adequate.

What harm can your treatment cause?

Some patients with COPD will be CO_2 retainers, requiring mild hypoxia to stimulate the respiratory center. An FIO_2 of 28% may remove this "hypoxic" drive to breathe. Unless there is or has been hypercarbia (check the old chart) it is difficult to predict which patients with COPD will be CO_2 retainers, and it is therefore

Table 20–1. DISCRIMINATING FEATURES IN THE HISTORY AND
PHYSICAL EXAMINATION OF A PATIENT WITH SOB

	CHF	Pulmonary Embolism and Infarction	Pneumonia	Asthma/ COPD
History				
Onset	Gradual	Sudden	Gradual	Gradual
Other	Orthopnea PND	Risk factors (see page 208)	Cough Fever Sputum production	Previous history
Physical Examination				
Temperature	Normal	Normal or slightly elevated	High	Normal
Pulsus parodoxus	No	No	No	Yes
JVP	Elevated	Elevated or normal	Normal	Normal
S_3	Present	Occasional RVS_3 present	Absent	Absent
Respiratory				
Crackles	Bibasal	Unilateral	Unilateral	
Wheezes	±	±	±	Present
Friction rub	No	±	±	No
Other	Pleural effusions		Consolidation Bronchial breath sounds Whispering pectoriloquy	

prudent to assume that all patients with COPD and heavy smoking histories are CO_2 retainers.

Administering 100% O_2 can cause atelectasis or O_2 toxicity if given over a period of days. This is of more concern in the mechanically ventilated patient, as these FIO_2 levels are impossible to attain unless the patient is intubated.

Why is the patient SOB or hypoxic?

There are four common causes of SOB in hospitalized patients, as follows:

Cardiovascular causes   1. CHF
                                 2. Pulmonary embolism
Pulmonary causes   3. Pneumonia
                                 4. Bronchospasm (asthma/COPD)

In most cases you will find it easy to distinguish among these four conditions. Look for specific associated signs and symptoms as outlined in Table 20–1 that will help you identify which one of the four major causes of SOB your patient is most likely to have and treat him or her accordingly. Once you have established which pattern of SOB your patient most likely has, take a more thorough selective history and physical examination.

Cardiovascular Causes: Congestive Heart Failure (CHF)

Selective History

- Is there a history of CHF or cardiac disorder?
- Is there orthopnea?
- Is there PND?
- Are there trends in daily weight or fluid balance records that may heighten your suspicion of fluid retention and hence CHF?

Selective Physical Examination
Assess the *volume status*. **Is the patient volume overloaded?**

VITALS	Tachycardia, tachypnea
HEENT	Elevated JVP
RESP	Inspiratory crackles $\pm$ pleural effusions (more often on the right side)
	Wheezes are suggestive of asthma but also may be seen in CHF.
CVS	Cardiac apex displaced laterally
	S_3
	Systolic murmurs (aortic stenosis, mitral regurgitation, VSD, tricuspid regurgitation)
	Diastolic murmurs (aortic regurgitation, mitral stenosis)
ABD	Hepatomegaly with positive HJR
EXT	Presacral or ankle edema
	Crackles and S_3 are the most reliable indicators of left-sided heart failure, while elevated JVP, enlarged liver, positive HJR, and peripheral edema indicate right-sided heart failure.

CXR (Fig. 20–2)

- Cardiomegaly
- Perihilar congestion
- Bilateral interstitial (early) or alveolar (more advanced) infiltrates
- Redistribution of pulmonary vasculature
- Kerley's B lines
- Pleural effusions

Treatment

General Measures

- IV D5W TKVO. IV access is required to deliver medications. Switch to a heparin lock when the acute episode has resolved.

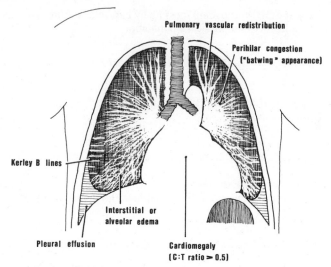

Figure 20–2. Chest x-ray features of congestive heart failure.

- O$_2$
- Restricted sodium diet
- Bed rest
- SC heparin (5000 U SC q12h)
- Fluid balance charting
- Daily weight

Specific Measures

Cardiac function can be improved by altering preload, afterload, or contractility. In the acute situation, all of your intervention will involve decreasing the preload.

- Sit the patient up; this position pools blood in the legs.
- *Morphine sulfate* 2 to 4 mg IV q5 to 10 min up to 10 to 12 mg pools blood in the splanchnic circulation. Morphine sulfate may cause hypotension or respiratory depression. Take the BP and RR before and after each dose is given. If necessary, *naloxone hydrochloride* 0.2 to 2.0 mg IV, IM, or SC may be used to reverse the hypotension or respiratory depression of morphine, up to a total of 10 mg. Nausea or vomiting may also occur and can usually be controlled with *dimenhydrinate* (Dramamine, Gravol) 25 mg IV or 50 mg PO/IM q4h PRN.
- *Nitroglycerin ointment* (Nitrol) 2.5 to 5.0 cm (1 to 2″) topically q4h. If nitroglycerin ointment is not readily available, you may instead give *nitroglycerin tablets* 0.3 to 0.6 mg SL or *nitroglycerin spray* one puff q15 min until the patient feels less SOB, as long as the systolic BP remains above 90 mm Hg. All nitroglycerin

preparations pool blood in the peripheral circulation. Nitroglycerin preparations commonly cause headaches. These can be treated with *acetaminophen* (Tylenol) 325 to 650 mg PO q4h PRN.

These three measures are temporary, shifting the excessive intravascular volume from the central veins. Only the diuretics actually reduce extracellular volume.

- *Furosemide* (Lasix) 40 mg IV given over 2 to 5 minutes. If there is no response (e.g., a lessening of the symptoms and signs of CHF, a diuresis) double the dose q1h (i.e., 40-80-160 mg) to a total dose of about 400 mg. Larger initial doses (e.g., 80-120 mg) may be required if the patient has renal insufficiency, is in severe CHF, or is already on maintenance furosemide. Doses of furosemide greater than 100 mg should be infused at a rate not exceeding 4 mg/min to avoid ototoxicity. Smaller initial doses (e.g., 10 mg) may suffice for frail, elderly (90-year-old) patients.
- If furosemide is ineffective try *ethacrynic acid* (Edecrin) 50 mg IV q60 min × 2 doses or *bumetanide* (Bumex) 1 to 10 mg IV over 1 to 2 minutes. (Bumex is a "loop diuretic" with a potency 40× that of furosemide.) *Furosemide, ethacrynic acid, and bumetanide* may cause hypokalemia, which is of particular concern in the digitalized patient. Monitor serum potassium level once or twice daily in the acute situation. High doses of these diuretics may also lead to serious sensorineural hearing loss, especially if the patient is also receiving other ototoxic agents, such as aminoglycoside antibiotics.

If diuretics are ineffective, it is unlikely that the patient is going to produce urine. Other methods of removing intravascular volume, such as *phlebotomy* (200 to 300 ml) and *rotating tourniquets,* are seldom required in the hospital setting. If there is a persistent component of bronchospasm ("cardiac asthma") an inhaled beta agonist or IV theophylline preparation may improve oxygenation.

Digoxin is not of benefit acutely unless the CHF has been precipitated by a bout of supraventricular tachycardia (e.g., rapid atrial fibrillation or flutter) which can be slowed by digoxin. (Refer to Chapter 12 for the management of tachydysrhythmias).

CHF is a symptom and a very serious one! After you have treated the symptom, sit down and ascertain *why* the patient developed CHF. This requires you to identify the *etiologic factor* of which there are six possibilities:

1. Myocardial infarction
2. Hypertension
3. Valvular heart disease
4. Congenital heart disease
5. Pericardial disease
6. Cardiomyopathy (dilated, restrictive, hypertrophic)

If the patient has a *history* of CHF the *etiologic factor* may already be identified for you in the patient's chart. However, the job does not end there, for now you must also identify a *precipitating factor* of which the following ten are most common:

1. Pulmonary embolism
2. Noncompliance with diet or medication
3. Cardiac depressant drugs (e.g., beta blockers, disopyramide, calcium entry blockers)
4. Sodium retaining agents (e.g., NSAIDs)
5. Increased sodium load (dietary, medicinal, parenteral)
6. Dysrhythmias
7. Renal disease
8. Anemia
9. Fever, infection
10. Pregnancy

Remember, that any **new** *etiologic factor* may also act as a *precipitating factor* in a patient with a history of CHF. Document the suspected *etiologic* and *precipitating* factors in the chart.

Cardiovascular Causes: Pulmonary Embolism

The classic triad of SOB, hemoptysis, and chest pain actually occurs in only a minority of cases. The best way to avoid missing this diagnosis is to consider it in each case of SOB you see.

Selective History
Look for predisposing causes.

Stasis

- Prolonged bed rest
- Immobilized limb
- Obesity
- CHF
- Pregnancy

Vein injury

- Trauma (especially hip fractures)
- Surgery (especially abdominal, pelvic, and orthopedic procedures)

Hypercoagulability

- Malignancy
- Inflammatory bowel disease
- Nephrotic syndrome

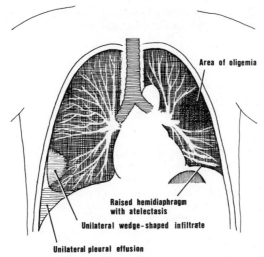

Figure 20–3. Variable chest x-ray features of pulmonary embolism.

- Use of birth control pills
- Deficiencies of antithrombin III, protein C or S

Selective Physical Examination

Features suggestive of pulmonary embolism include the following:

- Pleural friction rub
- Pulmonary consolidation
- Unilateral or bilateral pleural effusions
- Unilateral or bilateral wheeze
- Sudden onset cor pulmonale
- New onset tachydysrhythmia
- Simultaneous deep vein thrombosis (DVT)

CXR (Fig. 20–3)

- Atelectasis (loss of volume)
- Unilateral wedge-shaped pulmonary infiltrate
- Unilateral pleural effusion
- Raised hemidiaphragm
- Areas of oligemia
- Entirely normal

ECG

Only a massive pulmonary embolism will give you the classic right ventricular strain pattern of S_1, Q_3, right axis deviation, and

RBBB. The most common ECG finding is a *sinus tachycardia,* but other supraventricular tachycardias also may occur.

ABGs

The most common finding on ABG determination is acute respiratory alkalosis. Of patients with pulmonary embolism, 85% have $Po_2 < 80$ mm Hg on room air. If the Po_2 is > 80 mm Hg and pulmonary embolism is still suspected, look for an elevated $P(A-a)o_2$. (See Appendix for calculation.)

Management

If your suspicion for pulmonary embolism is high, you are obligated to begin anticoagulation without further confirmation of the diagnosis at this point. *However, prior to ordering heparin, ensure that the patient has no history of bleeding disorders, peptic ulcers, and intracranial disease, e.g., recent stroke, subarachnoid hemorrhage (SAH), tumor, and recent surgery;* all are contraindications to anticoagulation. These patients will require confirmation of pulmonary embolism with V/Q scan or pulmonary angiography and, if embolism is documented, consultation with a vascular surgeon for possible interruption of the inferior vena cava.

If there are *no contraindications* draw a blood sample for CBC, aPTT, and platelet count immediately. Begin *heparin* 100 units/kg IV bolus (usual dose = 5000 to 10,000 units IV) and follow with maintenance infusion of 1000 units/hr IV.

Heparin should be delivered by infusion pump, with maintenance dosing ordered as follows: heparin 25,000 units/500 ml D5W to run at 20 ml/hr = 1000 units/hr. It is dangerous to put large doses of heparin in small volume IV bags as "run-away" IVs filled with heparin can result in serious overdose.

Heparin and warfarin are dangerous drugs because of their potential for causing bleeding disorders. Write and double check your heparin orders carefully. Also, measure platelet counts once or twice a week to detect reversible heparin-induced thrombocytopenia which may occur at any time while a patient is on heparin.

After starting heparin obtain a V/Q scan as soon as possible to confirm diagnosis of pulmonary embolism. A *high probability* V/Q scan is sufficient evidence to continue anticoagulation. A *normal* V/Q scan rules out pulmonary embolism. A *low* or *intermediate* probability V/Q scan in the presence of high clinical suspicion should be confirmed by pulmonary angiography before committing the patient to long-term anticoagulation. Alternatively, demonstration of a simultaneous DVT by nuclear or contrast venography or impedance plethysmography is sufficient evidence to continue anticoagulation.

Monitor aPTT q6h and adjust heparin maintenance dose until aPTT is in the therapeutic range (1.5 to 2.0 times normal). After this, daily aPTTs are sufficient. Initial measurements of aPTT are made only to ensure adequate anticoagulation.

Continue IV heparin for 7 to 10 days. Add oral *warfarin* (Coumadin) within 3 days of starting heparin, beginning at 5 to 10 mg PO daily and titrating the dose to achieve a PT 1.2 to 1.5 times control. (Measure aPTT *and PT* daily during this initial adjustment phase.) Attainment of a therapeutic PT will usually take 5 to 6 days, after which the heparin can be discontinued.

Numerous drugs interfere with warfarin metabolism to increase or decrease the PT. Before prescribing *any* drug to a patient on warfarin, look up its effect on warfarin metabolism and monitor PTs carefully, if an interaction is anticipated.

Write an order that the patient should receive no aspirin or aspirin products and no IM injections while on anticoagulation.

Ask your patient daily about signs of bleeding or bruising. Instruct your patient that prolonged pressure after venipuncture will be required to prevent local bruising while on anticoagulation.

Pulmonary Causes: Pneumonia

Selective History and Physical Examination

- Cough productive of purulent sputum
- Fever
- Pleuritic chest pain
- Pulmonary consolidation ± pleural effusion

CXR

Variable findings from patchy diffuse infiltrates to consolidation ± pleural effusion. Remember that a volume depleted patient may not manifest the typical CXR findings of pneumonia until the intravascular volume is restored to normal. Trust your clinical examination.

Identify the Organism

- Sputum Gram's stain and culture. If the patient is not able to spontaneously cough up sputum you may induce it with ultrasonic nebulization or chest physiotherapy. Take a sputum sample to the laboratory yourself and examine the Gram's stain. (See Appendix for interpretation of the Gram's stain.)
- Blood culture (×2)
- Thoracentesis. Moderate to large pleural effusions should be tapped to exclude empyema. Pleural biopsy will also be necessary if TB is a consideration. Send pleural fluid to the laboratory for
- Gram's stain and aerobic and anaerobic cultures
- ZN stain and TB cultures
- Cell count and differential
- LDH
- Protein
- Glucose

If appropriate send for

- Fungal cultures
- pH
- Cytology
- Amylase
- Triglycerides

A simultaneous serum glucose, protein, and LDH should be drawn immediately after the pleural tap has been completed. These serum determinations are necessary to compare with pleural fluid values in assessing whether the fluid is a transudate or exudate.

Always consider TB in your differential diagnosis. Order ZN stains and sputum for culture if TB is suspected.

Management

General Measures

- O$_2$
- Chest physiotherapy

Specific Measures

- Antimicrobials

Your choice will depend on the Gram's stain results. If no sputum is available, several "rules of thumb" will help you out:

Outpatient acquired pneumonia in the non-immunocompromised host—*Streptococcus pneumoniae, Mycoplasma pneumoniae, Legionella pneumophila* (in some geographic locations). *Penicillin G* 1 to 2 million units IV q4 to 6h should be used in the patient suspected of having a pneumococcal pneumonia. Otherwise, a good antibacterial choice is *erythromycin* 500 mg PO or IV q6h.

Administration of erythromycin is painful and can cause thrombophlebitis when given intravenously. This can be minimized by diluting each 500 mg dose in 500 ml IV fluid and administering slowly over 6 hours. If volume overload is a concern each 500 mg dose can be added to 250 ml IV fluid and given over 6 hours.

Chronic obstructive pulmonary disease (COPD)—*S. pneumoniae, Haemophilus influenzae*. *Ampicillin* 1 gm PO or IV q6h is a good choice.

Aspiration pneumonias should be considered in any situation in which a decreased level of consciousness or an interference with the cough reflex has occurred (e.g., alcoholism, stroke, seizure, post-surgery). Episodes of aspiration do not require antibiotic treatment unless there are clinical signs of bacterial infection (fever, sputum production, leukocytosis). Aspirations acquired prior to hospital admission involve mouth anaerobes and can be treated with *penicillin G* 1 million units IV q6h or *clindamycin* 300 to 600 mg PO or IV q6h. Hospital-acquired aspirations should also be treated using gram-negative coverage (e.g., gentamicin).

Elderly (> 65 years of age) or *institutionalized* patients have an increased frequency of gram-negative pneumonias. A good choice for therapy is *cefazolin* (Ancef) 1 to 2 gm IV q8h ± an aminoglycoside.

Hospital-acquired pneumonias also require gram-negative coverage with a cephalosporin or an aminoglycoside until culture and sensitivity results are available. *Pseudomonas* and *Acinetobacter* are common ICU/CCU pathogens and can be treated by utilizing the known local antimicrobial sensitivities of these organisms in your hospital.

Alcoholics, in addition to aspiration pneumonias, have a high frequency of *Klebsiella pneumoniae.* This should be treated with two drugs—usually a cephalosporin and an aminoglycoside, e.g., *cefazolin* (Ancef) 1 to 2 gm IV q8h and *gentamicin* 1.5 to 2 mg/kg IV loading dose, followed with 1 to 1.5 mg/kg IV q8h of gentamicin if renal function is normal. Aminoglycosides can cause nephrotoxicity and ototoxicity.

Avoid these side effects by following serum aminoglycoside levels, usually after the third or fourth maintenance dose, and serum creatinine levels. If the patient already has renal insufficiency *give the same loading dose* but adjust the maintenance dose interval according to the creatinine clearance (see page 296, Appendix).

The most common infecting pulmonary pathogen in *AIDS patients* is *Pneumocystis carinii.* Urgent diagnostic bronchoscopy is advisable when this organism is suspected. If the patient looks sick and bronchoscopy is not immediately available, the attending physician may want you to give one dose of *trimethoprim-sulfamethoxasole* or *pentamidine isethionate* and arrange for bronchoscopy as soon as possible. Steroids may also be helpful in patients who are particularly ill with *P. carinii* pneumonia.

Pentamidine has numerous side effects including hypotension, tachycardia, nausea, vomiting, unpleasant taste, and flushing. Some of these side effects can be minimized by administering the dose in 500 ml D5W over 2 to 4 hours. In addition, biochemical abnormalities may include hyperkalemia; hypocalcemia; megaloblastic anemia; leukopenia; thrombocytopenia; hyperglycemia or hypoglycemia; elevated liver enzyme levels; and dose-related, reversible nephrotoxicity.

Pulmonary Causes: Bronchospasm (Asthma and COPD)

Asthma is a condition characterized by airflow obstruction that varies significantly over time.

Chronic obstructive pulmonary disease (COPD) may take the form of *chronic bronchitis,* which is a clinical diagnosis (production of mucoid sputum on most days for 3 months of the year in 2 consecutive years) or *emphysema,* which is a pathologic diagnosis (enlargement of airways distal to the terminal bronchioles). Most patients with COPD have features of both.

Selective History

- Does the patient smoke cigarettes?
- Is the patient on theophylline or steroids?
- Has the patient ever been intubated?
- Can precipitating factors (e.g., specific allergies, nonspecific irritants, URTI, pneumonia, beta blocker administration) be identified?
- Is the patient having an anaphylactic reaction?
  Look for evidence of systemic autocoid (e.g., histamine) release, i.e., wheezing, itch (urticaria), and hypotension. Anaphylactic reactions in hospitalized patients are most commonly seen after administration of IV dye, penicillin, or aspirin. If there is suspicion of anaphylaxis, refer immediately to Chapter 15, page 134, for appropriate management. This is an emergency!

Selective Physical Examination
Is there evidence of obstructive airways disease?

VITALS	Pulsus paradoxus
HEENT	Cyanosis
	Elevated JVP (cor pulmonale)
	Cor pulmonale is defined as right-sided heart failure secondary to pulmonary disease.
	Position of trachea
	A pneumothorax may be a complication of asthma/COPD and results in a shift of the trachea away from the affected side.
RESP	Intercostal in-drawing
	Use of accessory muscles of respiration
	Increased A/P diameter
	Hyperinflated lungs with depressed hemidiaphragms
	Wheezing
	Diffuse wheezing is most often a manifestation of asthma or COPD but may also be seen in CHF ("cardiac asthma"), pulmonary embolism, pneumonia, or anaphylactic reactions. Ensure that the patient has not undergone IV dye studies within the last 12 hours.
	Prolonged expiratory phase
CVS	Loud P_2
	RV heave, RVS_3 (pulmonary hypertension, cor pulmonale)

CXR

- Hyperinflation of lung fields
- Flattened diaphragms
- Increased A-P diameter
- Look also for infiltrates—suggesting concomitant pneumonia; atelectasis—suggesting mucous plugging; pneumothorax; or pneumomediastinum.

Management

General Measures

- O_2
- Hydration

Specific Measures

Step 1. Inhaled beta agonists, such as *salbutamol* (Ventolin) 2.5 to 5.0 mg in 3 ml NS by nebulizer q4h, *fenoterol* (Berotec) 0.5 to 1.0 mg in 3 ml NS by nebulizer q4 to 6h, or *orciprenaline* [metaproterenol] (Alupent) 0.2 to 0.3 ml in 2.5 ml NS by nebulizer q4h.

Although standard dosing intervals for beta agonists are q4 to 6h, they may be given almost continuously in severe bronchospasm, as long as you watch closely for potential side effects (supraventricular tachycardias, PVCs, muscle tremors).

Step 2. Theophylline preparation in patients not receiving theophylline in the last 24 hours. *Aminophylline* 6 mg/kg IV loading dose over 20 minutes, followed by maintenance dosage of 0.6 mg/kg/hr IV infusion. Give 0.3 mg/kg/hr in patients with CHF or liver disease and elderly patients and 0.9 mg/kg/hr in smokers. If the patient has received a theophylline-containing preparation in the past 24 hours, administer half the recommended loading dose, then follow with a full maintenance dose as previously recommended.

The therapeutic serum range for theophylline is 30 to 100 mmol/L. Higher levels cause cardiac stimulation (tachycardia, PVCs), GI upset (nausea, vomiting), and CNS irritability (headache, seizures). Remember that theophylline clearance is decreased by the addition of erythromycin, cimetidine (but usually not ranitidine), propranolol, allopurinol, and a number of other drugs.

Step 3. Steroids, e.g., *hydrocortisone* 250 mg IV bolus, followed by maintenance dose of 100 mg IV q6h. (Optimal steroid preparation and dosage is controversial). Remember that steroids take 6 hours to work, so they must be given now if persistent wheezing is anticipated in the next 6 to 24 hours. Beclomethasone dipropionate (Beclovent) is not useful in acute bronchospasm.

Steroids have few side effects in the short-term situation. Sodium retention is of concern in the patient with CHF or hypertension; hyperglycemia may occur in diabetics.

There has been a great deal of concern about tapering steroids too rapidly. A person on IV steroids for less than 2 weeks can have the steroids discontinued abruptly without fear of steroid withdrawal. Of more concern is exacerbation of wheezing as steroids are tapered; this may limit the rate at which steroids can be withdrawn.

When a patient develops an exacerbation of bronchospasm a general rule of thumb is to administer medications *one step beyond* what is usually required as an outpatient. For example, a patient normally controlled on a salbutamol inhaler at home will probably require both nebulized beta agonist and IV aminophylline during an exacerbation. If the patient is wheezing despite out-patient treatment with a beta agonist and a theophylline preparation or if the patient is already on a small dose of prednisone, then he or she should be given IV steroids during the acute attack. In the severe asthmatic, nebulized atropine or ipratropium may also be helpful.

Look for evidence of bronchitis or pneumonia as the precipitant of bronchospasm. In patients so affected, bronchospasm may persist until appropriate *antibiotics* are given.

Five Warning Signs in Asthma

1. Sudden acute deterioration in an asthmatic patient may represent a *pneumothorax*.
2. "Rising P_{CO_2}": Patients with an acute attack of asthma hyperventilate. A "normal" P_{CO_2} of 40 mm Hg in the acute situation may signify impending respiratory failure.
3. *Disappearance of wheezing*: In the acute situation this is an ominous sign, indicating that the patient is not moving enough air in and out to generate a wheeze.
4. *Sedatives are contraindicated in asthma and COPD.* The RN may not be aware of this and may unknowingly request a sleeping pill from your colleague while you are off duty. To avoid this pitfall, write clearly in your orders "No sedatives or sleeping pills."
5. Approximately 10% of asthmatic patients have a triad of asthma, nasal polyps, and aspirin sensitivity. When prescribing analgesics in asthmatics it is best to *avoid NSAIDs,* including aspirin, as fatal anaphylactoid reactions have occurred in some patients given these medications.

RESPIRATORY FAILURE

Any of the four conditions causing SOB and a variety of others may lead to respiratory failure. Suspect that this is occurring if the RR is less than 12/min or if there is thoracoabdominal dissociation. Confirm the diagnosis of acute respiratory failure by ABG determination. A Po_2 of < 50 mm Hg or a $Pco_2 > 50$ mm Hg with a pH < 7.30 while breathing room air indicates *acute respiratory failure*.

1. Ensure that the patient has not received narcotic analgesics in the last 24 hours, which may depress the RR. Pupillary constriction may give you a hint that a narcotic is the culprit. If a narcotic has been given or if you are uncertain order *naloxone hydrochloride* (Narcan) 0.2 to 2.0 mg IV immediately.

2. If no reponse to naloxone occurs, arrange for transfer of the patient to the ICU/CCU. Acute respiratory acidosis with pH < 7.30 *may* respond to aggressive treatment of the underlying respiratory or neuromuscular disorder but make arrangements for possible endotracheal intubation, if there is not rapid improvement. Acute respiratory acidosis with pH < 7.20 usually requires mechanical ventilation until the precipitating cause of respiratory deterioration can be reversed.

REMEMBER

1. Abdominal problems can masquerade as SOB. (One of us (SM) was once called to see a patient whose SOB resolved as soon as urinary retention was relieved by placement of a Foley's catheter and 1300 ml of urine was drained.) Massive ascites and obesity may also compromise respiratory function.

2. Do not be worried about your inexperience with endotracheal intubation. A patient in respiratory failure can be "bagged and masked" effectively for hours until someone with intubation experience is available to assist you.

3. Notice that *epinephrine* does not appear in the protocol for treatment of asthma. There is no need to use epinephrine in the adult with an attack of asthma or COPD unless bronchospasm as a component of an anaphylactic reaction is present. Epinephrine given inadvertently in cases of "cardiac asthma" has resulted in fatal MI.

21

SKIN RASHES AND URTICARIA

This chapter will not transform you into a dermatologist, able to diagnose any rash with one quick glance. It will, however, help you to describe accurately rashes for which you are called at night. This ability will facilitate confirmation of the diagnosis in the morning by more experienced physicians. Urticarial rashes are rare in hospitalized patients; however, they are important to recognize since they may be the prodrome of anaphylactic shock.

PHONE CALL

Questions

1. **How long has the patient had the rash?**
2. **Is there any urticaria (hives)?**
3. **Is there any audible wheezing or SOB?**
4. **What are the vital signs?**
5. **What drugs has the patient received within the past 12 hours?**
6. **Has the patient received IV contrast material within the past 12 hours?**
   Remember that patients receiving CT scans are often given IV contrast material.
7. **Does the patient have any known allergies?**
8. **What was the reason for admission?**

Orders

If the patient has evidence of anaphylaxis (urticaria, wheezing, SOB, or hypotension) order the following to be available at the bedside immediately:

1. IV to be started immediately with NS.
2. *Epinephrine* 5 ml (0.5 mg) of 1:10,000 for IV administration (this is available in a pre-drawn syringe from the emergency cart) or *epinephrine* 0.5 ml (0.5 mg) of 1:1000 for SC administration. Epinephrine may be required *either* IV *or* SC depending upon the severity of the reaction. Do not confuse these doses and routes of administration.
3. Diphenhydramine (Benadryl) 50 mg IV.
4. Hydrocortisone (Solu-Cortef) 250 mg IV.

Inform RN

"Will arrive at bedside in . . . minutes."

Evidence of anaphylaxis (urticaria, wheezing, SOB, or hypotension) requires you to see the patient immediately. Assessment of a skin rash, with no associated symptoms of anaphylaxis, can wait an hour or two if other problems of higher priority exist.

ELEVATOR THOUGHTS (What Causes Skin Rashes?)

The majority of calls at night regarding skin rashes are due to drug eruptions. The lesions may be urticarial, which is rare but potentially life-threatening; erythematous; vesicular; bullous; or purpuric. The distribution of the rash is usually generalized except for "fixed drug eruptions" (see following section).

Causes of Urticaria: Rare but Life-threatening

Drugs Causing Release of Histamine

- IV contrast material
- Opiates (codeine, morphine, meperidine)
- Antibiotics (penicillins, cephalosporins, sulfonamides, tetracycline, quinine, polymyxin, isoniazid)
- Anesthetic agents (curare)
- Vasoactive agents (atropine, amphetamine, hydralazine)
- Miscellaneous (bile salts, thiamine, dextran, deferoxamine)

Drugs (Mechanism Unclear)

- Aspirin and other NSAIDs

Hereditary Angioedema

Food Allergies Causing Histamine Release

- Fruits, tomatoes, lobster, shrimp

Physical Agents

- Dermatographia, cold, heat, pressure, vibration

Idiopathic

Erythematous, Maculopapular (Morbilliform) Rashes

- Antibiotics (penicillin, ampicillin, sulfonamides, chloramphenicol)

- Antihistamines
- Anti-depressants (amitriptylline)
- Diuretics (thiazides)
- Oral hypoglycemics
- Anti-inflammatory drugs (gold, phenylbutazone)
- Sedatives (barbiturates)

Ampicillin commonly causes a generalized maculopapular eruption 2 to 4 weeks after administration of the first dose. Thus, it is important to check not only the current drugs the patient is receiving but also all recently discontinued drugs, since the eruption may appear several weeks after the drug has been stopped.

Vesicobullous Rashes

- Antibiotics (sulfonamides, dapsone)
- Anti-inflammatory drugs (penicillamine)
- Sedatives (barbiturates)
- Halogens (iodides, bromides)

Purpura

- Antibiotics (sulfonamides, chloramphenicol)
- Diuretics (thiazides)
- Anti-inflammatory drugs (phenylbutazone, indomethacin, salicylates)

Drug-induced thrombocytopenia causes non-palpable purpura, whereas vasculitis causes palpable purpura.

Exfoliative Dermatitis (Erythroderma)

- Antibiotics (streptomycin)
- Anti-inflammatory drugs (gold, phenylbutazone)
- Anti-epileptics (carbamazepine)

If a drug eruption is not recognized early and the drug is not discontinued, the patient may develop a generalized, dusky red, dry rash with profound scaling.

Fixed Drug Eruption

- Antibiotics (sulfonamides, metronidazole)
- Anti-inflammatory drugs (phenylbutazone)
- Analgesics (phenacetin)
- Sedatives (barbiturates, chlordiazepoxide)
- Laxatives (phenolphthalein)

Certain drugs may produce a skin lesion in a specific area. Repeat administration of the drug reprodces the skin lesion in the same location. The lesion is usually dusky red patches distributed over the trunk or proximal limbs.

MAJOR THREAT TO LIFE

■ Anaphylactic shock

Urticarial skin rash may be a prodrome of anaphylaxis; other types of skin rashes are not. Drugs and IV contrast material are the usual causes of anaphylactic shock in hospitalized patients—unless the patient was unlucky enough to be stung by a wasp or to have eaten shrimp.

BEDSIDE

Quick Look Test

Does the patient look well (comfortable), sick (uncomfortable or distressed), or critical (about to die)?
The patient with an anaphylactic reaction looks apprehensive and, unless moribund, is usually SOB and sitting up in bed.

Airway and Vital Signs

What is the BP?
Hypotension is an ominous sign in anaphylactic shock, and the patient requires immediate treatment. If anaphylaxis is suspected, insert a large bore IV (#16 when possible), if not already done, and run in NS as fast as possible.

What is the temperature?
Skin rashes are often more prominent when the patient is febrile.

Selective Physical Examination

Is there evidence of an impending anaphylactic reaction?

HEENT Pharyngeal, periorbital, or facial edema (anaphylaxis)
RESP   Audible wheezing or high-pitched wheezing (anaphylaxis)
       If evidence of an impending anaphylactic reaction exists, refer to page 134 for immediate treatment.
SKIN   When an urticarial rash appearing as a manifestation of anaphylaxis has been ruled out, the remaining task is to describe the rash accurately to help you diagnose the lesion and perhaps to help someone else diagnose it, if it disappears or changes by the morning.

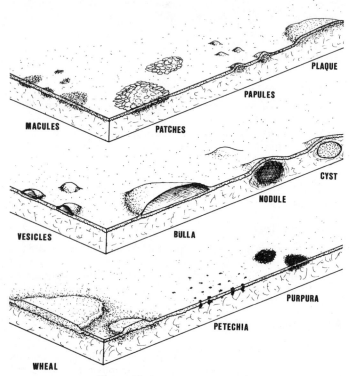

Figure 21-1. Primary skin lesions.

Describe the Location of the Rash
Is it generalized, acral (hands, feet), or localized?

The location of the rash is one of the most helpful features enabling you to narrow the diagnostic possibilities.

Describe the Color of the Rash

■ Red, pink, brown, white

Describe the Primary Lesion (Fig. 21-1)

■ macule—flat (noticeable from the surrounding skin because of the color difference)
■ patch—macule with surface changes (scaling or wrinkling)
■ papule—solid, elevated, size < 1 cm
■ plaque—solid, elevated, size > 1 cm
■ vesicle—elevated, well circumscribed, size < 1 cm
■ bulla—elevated, well circumscribed, size > 1 cm

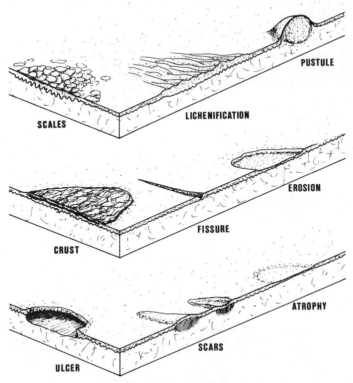

Figure 21–2. Secondary skin lesions.

- nodule—deep seated mass, indistinct borders, size < 0.5 cm in both width and depth
- cyst—nodule filled with expressible fluid or semi-solid material
- wheal—*hives*—well circumscribed, flat topped, firm elevation (papule, plaque, or dermal edema) ± central pallor, and irregular borders
- petechia—red-purple, non-blanchable macules, size < 3 mm
- purpura—red-purple, non-blanchable macules or papule, size > 3 mm

Describe the Secondary Lesion (Fig. 21–2)

- scales—dry, thin plates of thickened keratin layer (white color differentiates it from crust)
- lichenification—dry, leathery thickening, shiny surface, accentuated skin markings
- pustule—vesicle containing purulent exudate

- crust—dried, yellow exudate of plasma (result of broken vesicle, bulla, or pustule)
- fissure—linear, epidermal tear
- erosion—wide, epidermal fissure; moist and well circumscribed
- ulcer—erosion into the dermis
- scar—flat, raised, or depressed area of fibrosis
- atrophy—depression secondary to thinning of the skin

Describe the Configuration of the Rash

- annular—circular
- linear—in lines
- grouped—clusters, e.g., vesicular lesions of herpes zoster or herpes simplex

Selective History and Chart Review

- **How long has the rash been present?**
- **Does it itch?**
- **How has it been treated?**
- **Is this a new or a recurrent problem?**
- **Which drugs was the patient receiving before the rash started?**

Management

1. If the rash is associated with urticaria and thought to be secondary to a drug reaction, the drug should be withheld until confirmation of the diagnosis in the morning.
2. If the rash is non-urticarial and thought to be secondary to a drug reaction and the drug is deemed essential to the patient's management, the drug should be continued until confirmation of the diagnosis in the morning.
3. When the skin rash is not a drug eruption, and the diagnosis is clear, the standard recommended treatment can be instituted. (Refer to a dermatology text for specific treatment.)
4. Often house staff have difficulty in diagnosing skin rashes with any degree of certainty. If uncertain, it is sufficient to describe the lesion accurately and refer the patient to a dermatologist.

22

SYNCOPE

Syncope is a brief loss of consciousness due to sudden reduction in cerebral blood flow. A new term, "pre-syncope," has been coined referring to the situation in which there is reduction of cerebral blood flow sufficient to result in a sensation of impending loss of consciousness, though the patient does not actually "pass out." Pre-syncope and syncope represent degrees of the same disorder and should be addressed as manifestations of the same underlying problem. Your task is to discover the *cause* of the syncopal attack.

PHONE CALL

Questions

1. **Did the patient actually lose consciousness?**
2. **Is the patient still unconscious?**
3. **What are the vital signs?**
4. **Was the patient recumbent, sitting, or standing when the episode occurred?**
   Syncope while the patient is in the recumbent position is almost always cardiac in origin.
5. **Was any seizure-like activity witnessed?**
6. **What is the admitting diagnosis?**
   An admitting diagnosis of seizure disorder, transient ischemic attack, or cardiac disease may help direct you to the cause of the syncopal attack.
7. **Has the patient sustained any evidence of injury?**

Orders

If the patient is still *unconscious* order the following:

1. IV D5W TKVO immediately, if IV not already in place.
2. Turn the patient on the left side. This maneuver prevents the tongue from falling back into the throat, obstructing the upper airway, and also minimizes the risk of aspiration should vomiting occur.
3. Stat 12-lead ECG and rhythm strip. Though almost all patients with syncope will regain consciousness within a few minutes, you are more likely to be able to document a cardiac dysrhythmia early on while the patient is still symptomatic.

4. If the patient has *regained consciousness*, if there is no evidence of head or neck injury, and if the vital signs are stable do the following:
   a. In order to return the patient to bed, ask the RN to slowly raise the patient to a sitting position, then a standing position.
   b. The patient should be placed back in bed with the siderails up with instructions for the patient to remain in bed until you are able to assess the problem.
   c. Order an ECG and rhythm strip.
   d. Have the vital signs taken q15 min until you arrive at the bedside. Ask the RN to call you back immediately should the vital signs become unstable before you are able to assess the patient.

Inform RN

"Will arrive at bedside in . . . minutes."

Syncope requires you to see the patient immediately, if the patient is still unconscious or if there are abnormalities in the heart rate or blood pressure. If the patient is alert and conscious with normal vital signs (and if there are other more urgent problems to be assessed) the RN may observe the patient and call you if a problem arises before you are able to assess the patient.

ELEVATOR THOUGHTS (What causes syncope?)

Cardiac Causes

Dysrhythmias

Tachycardias	Ventricular tachycardia
	Ventricular fibrillation
Bradycardias	Sinus bradycardia
	Second- and third-degree AV block
	SSS

Pacemaker Syncope

- Pacemaker not working
- Pacemaker syndrome

Syncope with Exertion

- Aortic stenosis
- Asymmetric septal hypertrophy

Neurologic Causes

- Brain stem transient ischemic attack or stroke ("drop attacks")
- Seizure

- Subarachnoid hemorrhage

Vagal Causes

- The common "faint"
- Valsalva's maneuver
- Cough syncope
- Micturition syncope

Carotid Sinus Syncope

Orthostatic Hypotension

- Drug-induced
- Volume depletion
- Autonomic dysfunction

Miscellaneous

- Hyperventilation
- Anxiety attacks

MAJOR THREAT TO LIFE

If still unconscious, *aspiration*. If conscious, recurrence of potentially fatal cardiac *dysrhythmias*.

Since most patients recover from syncopal attacks within a few minutes, the actual loss of consciousness experienced by the patient is not the major problem. Of greater importance is that, while unconscious, the patient's tongue may block the oropharynx or the patient may aspirate oral or gastric contents into the lungs, an occurrence that may result in the development of aspiration pneumonia or ARDS. Therefore, in the unconscious patient, your primary goal is to protect the airway until the patient regains consciousness, and the cough reflexes are once again effective.

Once the patient has regained consciousness, the major threat to life is the recurrence of an unrecognized potentially fatal cardiac dysrhythmia. This can be best identified and managed by transferring the patient to an ICU/CCU or other setting with ECG monitors, if there is suspicion that a dysrhythmia was responsible for the syncopal episode.

BEDSIDE

Quick Look Test

Does the patient look well (comfortable), sick (uncomfortable or distressed), or critical (about to die)?

This simple observation helps determine the necessity of immediate intervention. Most patients who have had episodes of syncope and have regained consciousness look perfectly well.

Airway and Vital Signs

Airway. If the patient is still unconscious, ensure that the RN has placed him or her on the left side and that the patient's tongue has not fallen into the back of the throat. Most causes of syncope are very short lived, and by the time you arrive at the bedside the patient will have regained consciousness. Look for abnormalities in the vital signs, which may help make your diagnosis of the specific cause of syncope much easier.

What is the heart rate?

Supraventricular or ventricular tachycardia should be documented on ECG tracings, and the patient should be treated immediately. (Refer to Chapter 12, page 103, for treatment of supraventricular tachycardia and Chapter 12, page 105, for treatment of ventricular tachycardia).

Any patient with a transient or persistent supraventricular or ventricular tachycardia or its history when no other cause of syncope can be found should be transferred to the ICU/CCU or other setting with ECG monitoring for appropriate management.

What is the BP?

The patient with resting or orthostatic *hypotension* should be managed as outlined in Chapter 15. Remember that a massive internal hemorrhage, such as a GI bleed or a ruptured aortic aneurysm, occasionally can present with a syncopal attack.

Hypertension, if found in association with headache and neck stiffness, may indicate subarachnoid hemorrhage. A brief loss of consciousness is common at the onset of a subarachnoid hemorrhage and is often associated with dizziness, vertigo, or vomiting.

What is the temperature?

Patients with syncope are rarely febrile. If fever is present, it is usually due to a concomitant illness not related to the syncopal attack. However, especially if the syncopal attack was unwitnessed, be careful to exclude the possibility of a seizure secondary to meningitis, which may present as "fever and syncope."

Selective History and Chart Review

Has this ever happened before?

If it has, ask the patient if a diagnosis was made after the previous attack.

What do the patient or witnesses recall from the time immediately prior to the syncope?

- Syncope occurring while changing from the supine or sitting *position* to the standing position suggests orthostatic hypotension.
- An *aura*, though rare, is helpful in pointing to a seizure as the cause of syncope in an unwitnessed attack.
- *Palpitations* preceding an attack may suggest a cardiac dysrhythmia as a cause of syncope.
- Syncope during or immediately following performance of *Valsalva's* maneuver, a bout of *coughing*, or *micturition* may be due to mechanical reduction of venous return.
- Syncope after *turning the head to one side*, especially if one is wearing a tight collar, may represent carotid sinus syncope. This condition is most often seen in elderly men.
- Numbness and tingling in the hands and face are commonly seen just prior to the pre-syncope or syncope due to hyperventilation or anxiety.

Is there any history of cardiac disease?

A patient with pre-existing cardiac disease may have an increased risk of developing dysrhythmias.

Has the patient ever had a seizure?

An unwitnessed seizure may present as a syncopal attack. Ask the patient if during the attack he bit his tongue or if he were incontinent of stool or urine. Either one is suggestive of seizure activity.

Has the patient ever had a stroke?

A patient with known cerebrovascular disease is a likely candidate for a brain stem transient ischemic attack or stroke. However, remember that since atherosclerosis is a diffuse process, the patient with a history of stroke may also have coronary atherosclerosis that may result in cardiac dysrhythmias.

What does the patient remember upon waking from the syncopal attack?

Headache, drowsiness, and mental confusion are common sequelae of seizures but not of cardiac causes of syncope.

What are the medications?

Check the chart to see what medications the patient is being given.

Digoxin, propranolol, and calcium entry blockers may result in bradycardias. Digoxin, if present in toxic amounts, may also precipitate ventricular tachycardia.

Quinidine, procainamide, disopyramide, sotalol, amiodarone, tricyclic antidepressants, and phenothiazines may prolong the QT interval leading to ventricular tachycardia ("Torsades de pointes")

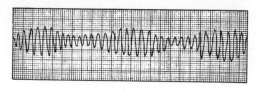

a

Prolonged Q-T interval
(usually ⟩ 0.40 s)

b

Figure 22–1. a = torsades de pointes and b = prolonged QT interval.

(Fig. 22–1A) or the "prolonged QT interval syndrome" (Fig. 22–1B).

Prazosin can occasionally cause syncope, if more than 2 mg is given as an initial dose.

Phenothiazines and tricyclic antidepressants lower the seizure threshold and may result in seizure.

Selective Physical Examination

Your physical examination is directed towards finding a cause for the syncope. However, a search for evidence of injuries sustained if the patient fell during the syncopal attack is equally important at this time.

VITALS   Repeat now.
HEENT   Fundoscopy—look for subhyaloid hemorrhages (SAH). Blood diffuses between the retinal fiber layer and the internal limiting membrane, forming a pocket of blood with sharp borders and often a fluid level.
          Tongue or cheek laceration (seizure disorder)
          Carotid or vertebrobasilar bruits (TIA or stroke). A vertebral artery bruit may sometimes be heard by listening with your stethoscope over the base of the

neck and may represent vertebrobasilar stenosis.
Neck stiffness (meningitis leading to a seizure; SAH)

RESP Crackles, wheezes (aspiration during the syncopal episodes)

CVS Pacemaker (pacemaker syncope)
Flat JVP (volume depletion)
Atrial fibrillation (vertebrobasilar embolism)
Systolic murmur (aortic stenosis; asymmetric septal hypertrophy)

GU Urinary incontinence (seizure disorder)
RECTAL Incontinence of stool (seizure disorder)
MSS Palpate bones for evidence of fracture that may have been sustained, if the patient fell.
NEURO A complete neurologic examination must be done looking for evidence of residual localizing signs that may indicate a space-occupying TIA, completed stroke, SAH, intracranial lesion, or Todd's paralysis. Vertebrobasilar TIAs or strokes are frequently accompanied by other evidence of brain stem dysfunction (e.g., cranial nerve abnormalities, such as diplopia, nystagmus, facial paralysis, vertigo, dysphagia, dysarthria).

Management

An immediate cause for syncope frequently cannot be found. Because treatment of the various causes of syncope is so different, one must have *documented proof* of the cause of a syncopal episode before proceeding to definitive treatment; investigations may take several days to complete. Your job, once you have assessed a patient with syncope, is to decide from the history, physical findings, and laboratory data what the most likely cause of syncope is and to arrange for further investigation, if necessary.

Cardiac Causes

If a cardiac cause of syncope is suspected, whether related to dysrhythmia, valvular, or pacemaker cause, the patient should be transferred to the CCU or to an intermediate care unit where continuous ECG monitoring is available. If there are no ECG monitored beds available and if there is no suspicion of ischemia-induced dysrhythmia, 24-hour Holter's monitoring should be arranged for the patient first thing in the morning.

Always consider a silent MI with subsequent transient AV block, ventricular tachycardia, or ventricular fibrillation as the cause for syncope of cardiac origin.

Treatment of specific dysrhythmias, if still present at the time you are assessing the patient, is discussed in Chapter 12.

Tachycardias	Ventricular tachycardia (page 105)
	Ventricular fibrillation (page 291)
Bradycardias	Sinus bradycardia (page 112)
	AV blocks (page 112)
	SSS (page 112)

Pacemaker syncope will require cardiologic consultation for replacement of the pacemaker or reprogramming of its pacing rate.

If *aortic stenosis* or *asymmetric septal hypertrophy* is thought to be responsible for exertional syncope, arrange for an ECG in the morning to document the suspected cardiac lesion and ask for a cardiologic consultation.

Neurologic Causes

Suspected *brain stem TIA or stroke* should be evaluated by a CT scan of the head. Anticoagulation or platelet inhibitors should be started only after consultation with a neurologist.

If a *seizure* is suspected you must first document the cause of the seizure as outlined in Chapter 19, page 189.

If an SAH is suspected, arrange for an urgent non-contrast CT scan of the head, looking for evidence of aneurysm or blood in the subarachnoid space. A normal CT scan does not, however, exclude an SAH, and an LP may be required to look for xanthochromic cerebrospinal fluid. If such a lesion is identified, a neurosurgeon should be consulted for further investigation and management.

Vagal Causes

Suspected vasovagal attacks can be managed without transfer to the ICU/CCU, as outlined in Chapter 15, page 131.

The definitive diagnosis of *carotid sinus syncope* requires potentially dangerous carotid sinus pressure, which must be done while the ECG is being monitored for cardiac dysrhythmias. Although the patient does not require ICU/CCU admission overnight, arrangements should be made in the morning to evaluate the cardiac rhythm during carotid sinus massage.

Orthostatic Hypotension

Syncope due to *volume depletion* can be managed with IV fluid replacement as outlined in Chapter 15, page 135.

Drug-induced orthostatic hypotension and *autonomic dysfunction* are complex treatment problems and, as long as the patient's volume status is normal, can be addressed in the morning through consultation with a neurologist or clinical pharmacologist.

Until the underlying problem responsible for orthostatic hypotension is corrected, instruct patients that if they must be out of bed during the night, they should (1) ask the RN for assistance and (2) move slowly from the supine to sitting position and then move slowly again from the sitting to standing position.

Miscellaneous

Syncope due to *hyperventilation* or *anxiety states* can be alleviated by instructing the patient to breathe into a paper bag when he or she begins to feel anxious or "pre-syncopal." This step will corrct hypocapnea and thereby prevent a syncopal attack.

REMEMBER

1. In the elderly patient, the main hazard of a syncopal attack is not necessarily an underlying disease but rather a fracture or other injury sustained during a fall.
2. Except for the Stokes-Adams attack (third-degree AV block), true syncope rarely occurs when a patient is in the recumbent position.

Blood transfusions are given around-the-clock in hospitals. Reactions to blood products may vary from the severe to the very mild. An organized approach will help you sort out both the nature of the reaction and what to do about it.

PHONE CALL

Questions

1. **What symptoms does the patient have?**
   Fever, chills, chest pain, back pain, diaphoresis, and SOB can all be manifestations of a transfusion reaction.
2. **What are the vital signs?**
3. **Which blood product is being transfused and how long ago was it started?**
4. **What was the reason for admission?**

Orders

1. Stop the transfusion immediately if the patient has any of the following symptoms:
   a. Sudden onset of hypotension
   b. Chest or back pain
   c. Any symptom (even fever, chills, or urticaria) occurring within minutes of the transfusion being started.
   d. Fever in a patient who has never before received a blood transfusion or who has never been pregnant. This symptom may represent an acute hemolytic reaction.

      An acute hemolytic transfusion reaction can appear with any of the aforementioned symptoms. Acute hemolytic reactions, although very rare, are associated with an extremely high mortality rate, which is proportionate to the volume of blood infused. In previously pregnant or transfused patients fever may be a non-hemolytic febrile reaction.
2. If the blood transfusion has been stopped, keep the IV open with NS.

Inform RN

"Will arrive at bedside in . . . minutes."

Any suspected hemolytic or anaphylactic transfusion reaction requires you to see the patient immediately.

ELEVATOR THOUGHTS (What causes transfusion reactions?)

Hemolytic Reactions

Immune Hemolysis

Mismatched RBCs (ABO incompatibility) are errors in either identification of the patient or labelling of the blood. Mismatched RBCs result in an acute hemolytic reaction; they are exceedingly rare and usually occur in emergency situations (i.e., in the post-anesthetic, operating, or emergency room), when the usual precautions in identification of the patient or labelling of the blood are breached. Delayed hemolytic reactions occur 3 to 14 days after transfusions and are due to trace amounts of alloantibodies to minor antigens from previous transfusions or pregnancies undetected by the crossmatch. Patients with these reactions present with low-grade fevers, anemia, and mild elevations in bilirubin levels.

Non-immune Hemolysis

Non-immune hemolysis may occur if the blood has been overheated or has undergone trauma. Trauma to blood products occurs either by excessive hand squeezing or pumping of the infusion bag during the rapid administration of blood in an emergency or by being delivered through too small a needle.

Anaphylaxis (IgG Response to IgA Antibodies)

Anaphylaxis may result from transmission of IgA antibodies from the donor's blood into a presensitized IgA-deficient patient.

Congenital IgA deficiency is a common (1:1000), asymptomatic disorder. The first transfusion that an IgA-deficient patient receives will contain IgA antibodies, which are recognized by the patient's immune system as foreign antigens. Thus, the IgA-deficient patient becomes sensitized and develops *anti-IgA antibodies*, which may result in anaphylaxis or urticaria with subsequent transfusions. There are two known IgA allotypes. (An allotype is simply a genetic variation in the structure of the immunoglobulin.)

Anaphylactic reactions are more common in patients who lack both allotypes of IgA, but they have been reported in patients who lack only one allotype. Individuals with IgA molecules of one allotype may develop antibodies against the other allotype, with subsequent transfusion reactions being exhibited as urticaria or, occasionally, anaphylaxis.

Urticaria

Transmission of the following antigens from the donor's blood can cause urticaria:

1. Food allergens, e.g., shrimp (IgE response)

2. Other plasma protein allergens
3. IgA antibodies into an IgA-deficient patient (i.e., deficient in one of the two allotypes). This is a very rare cause of urticaria.

Fever

1. Non-hemolytic febrile reaction
2. Early sign of acute hemolytic transfusion reaction. The patient's anti-HLA antibodies (from previous blood transfusions or pregnancies) react with the donor's WBCs, platelets, or both.
3. Pulmonary leukoagglutinin reaction. The donor's blood (usually from a multiparous woman) contains antibodies to the patient's WBCs, resulting in the agglutinated WBCs lodging in the pulmonary capillaries, causing non-cardiogenic pulmonary edema.
4. Microbial contamination (very rare). Although many infectious agents can be transmitted via blood transfusions (e.g., non-A, non-B hepatitis, malaria, syphilis, CMV, infectious mononucleosis, toxoplasmosis, rubella, Rocky Mountain spotted fever), they do not result in reactions during infusion of the blood product.

Blood banks in North America now screen for HIV and hepatitis B prior to blood being released for transfusion.

Pulmonary Edema

1. CHF. Volume overload may be induced in the patient with a history of CHF, since blood transfusions expand the intravascular volume.
2. Pulmonary leukoagglutinin reaction (see previous section).

MAJOR THREAT TO LIFE

- Acute hemolytic reaction
- Anaphylaxis

Both these reactions are very rare, but when they do occur, they can be fatal.

BEDSIDE

Quick Look Test

Does the patient look well (comfortable), sick (uncomfortable or distressed), or critical (about to die)?
The patient with impending anaphylaxis may look sick (agitated,

restless, or SOB). Patients with pulmonary edema secondary to a transfusion reaction may look critical, with severe SOB.

Airway and Vital Signs

What is the BP?

Hypotension is an ominous sign—ensure the transfusion has been stopped. It is seen in acute hemolytic reactions and in anaphylactic reactions. However, in the situation where the transfusion is being given for volume depletion, e.g., acute blood loss, hypotension may represent continued loss of intravascular volume from uncontrolled bleeding.

Tag and Wrist Band Check

Compare the identification tag on the blood with the patient's wrist band.

Selective Physical Examination

HEENT   Flushed face (hemolytic reaction or anaphylaxis)
         Pharyngeal, periorbital, or facial edema (anaphylaxis)
RESP   Wheezes (anaphylaxis)
NEURO   Decreased level of consciousness (anaphylaxis or hemolytic reaction)
SKIN   Heat along the vein being used for the transfusion (hemolytic reaction)
         Oozing from IV sites may be the only sign of hemolysis in the unconscious or anesthetized patient. DIC is a late manifestation of an acute hemolytic reaction.
URINE   Check the urine color
         Free Hb will turn urine red or brown and is indicative of a hemolytic reaction.

If there is evidence of anaphylaxis or hemolysis, *stop the transfusion* and immediately begin emergency treatment (see page 238).

Selective History

Ask again about symptoms that the patient may have developed since the initial phone call as follows:

- Fever or chills (non-hemolytic febrile reaction)
- Headache, chest pain, back pain, or diaphoresis (hemolytic reaction)
- SOB (volume overload or pulmonary leukoagglutinin reaction). A leukoagglutinin reaction occurring in the elderly patient is often misdiagnosed as cardiogenic pulmonary edema.

Has the patient had previous transfusion reactions? Chills and fever are most common in the patient who has received multiple transfusions or who has had several pregnancies.

Management

Anaphylaxis

1. Ensure the transfusion has been stopped.
2. *Epinephrine* 3 to 5 ml (0.3 to 0.5 mg) of 1:10,000 solution IV by slow, direct injection may repeat q5 minutes as necessary. If epinephrine 1:10,000 solution is not immediately available, it can be made by adding 1 ml of a 1:1000 solution to 9 ml of NS.
3. *NS* 500 to 1000 ml IV to be given as fast as possible through a "wide-open" IV.
4. *Oxygen* by bag and mask if necessary.
5. *Diphenhydramine* (Benadryl) 50 mg IV by slow, direct injection.
6. *Hydrocortisone* (Solu-Cortef) 250 mg IV by slow, direct injection.
7. Intubation if necessary.

Acute Hemolytic Reaction

1. Ensure the transfusion has been stopped.
2. NS 500 ml IV to be given as fast as possible.
   Try to maintain the urine output over 100 ml/hr with IV fluids and diuretics.
3. *Furosemide* (Lasix) 40 mg IV by slow, direct injection at a rate not faster than 4 mg/min or *mannitol* 25 gm IV over 5 minutes (to promote diuresis).
4. Draw 20 ml of the patient's blood and send for the following:
   a. Repeat crossmatch
   b. Coombs's test, free Hb
   c. CBC, RBC morphology
   d. Platelets, PT, aPTT, FDP
   e. Urea, creatinine levels
   f. Unclotted blood for a stat spin
      Hemolysis is demonstrated when the plasma remains pink despite spinning for 5 minutes (i.e., hemoglobinemia). This is a more rapid way of confirming hemoglobinemia than Coombs's test.
5. Obtain a urine sample for free Hb. In addition, urine can be tested with dipsticks in the unit. If there is hemoglobinuria, the dipstick results will be positive for Hb and negative for RBCs.
6. Send the donor's blood back to the blood bank for the following:
   a. Repeat crossmatch
   b. Coombs's test
7. If oliguria develops despite adequate IV fluids and appropriate diuretics, then *acute renal failure* should be suspected. (For management of acute renal failure, see Chapter 7, page 57).

Urticaria

1. Do not stop the transfusion. Hives alone are rarely serious but "hives and hypotension" is an anaphylactic reaction until proved otherwise.
2. *Diphenhydramine* (Benadryl) 50 mg PO or IV.
3. Prior to future transfusions, the patient should be premedicated with *diphenhydramine* 50 mg PO or IV (*not* IM). If this fails to prevent urticarial reactions, washed RBCs should be given.

Fever

1. Do not stop the transfusion unless a hemolytic reaction is suspected. Fever developing within minutes of a blood transfusion's being started is very likely to be a symptom of a hemolytic reaction.
2. Often no treatment is required. If the fever is high and the patient is distressed, however, an antipyretic drug may be ordered.
3. If the patient has documented fever with two consecutive blood transfusions, pre-medication with an antipyretic prior to subsequent transfusions is indicated. If this step fails to prevent fever, washed RBCs can be given.

Pulmonary Edema

1. Stop the transfusion or slow the rate of transfusion, unless the patient urgently needs blood.
2. *Furosemide* (Lasix) 40 mg IV. If the patient is already receiving a diuretic or if there is renal insufficiency, a higher dose of furosemide may be required.
3. For the management of CHF refer to Chapter 20, page 205. Volume overload, with subsequent pulmonary edema, should be anticipated in a patient with a history of CHF. This problem may be prevented by administering a diuretic (furosemide 40 mg IV) during the transfusion.

LABORATORY-RELATED PROBLEMS: FIVE COMMON CALLS

24

CALCIUM DISORDERS

HYPERCALCEMIA

Causes

1. Increased intake/absorption
   a. Vitamin D or A intoxication
   b. Excessive calcium supplementation
   c. Milk-alkali syndrome (excessive antacid ingestion)
   d. Sarcoidosis and other granulomatous diseases
2. Increased production/mobilization from bone
   a. Primary hyperparathyroidism
   b. Tertiary hyperparathyroidism. Primary parathyroid adenoma unmasked following renal transplantation.
   c. Neoplasm. There are four mechanisms for hypercalcemia of malignancy as follows:
      (1) Bony metastasis (prostate, thyroid, kidney, breast, lung, multiple myeloma)
      (2) PTH-like substance elaborated by tumor cells (lung, kidney, ovary, colon)
      (3) Prostaglandin E_2 increases bony reabsorption (multiple myeloma)
      (4) Osteoclast activating factor (multiple myeloma, lympho-proliferative disorders)
   d. Paget's disease
   e. Immobilization
   f. Hyperthyroidism
   g. Adrenal insufficiency
   h. Acromegaly
   i. Sarcoidosis. In addition to sarcoidosis increasing absorption from the GI tract, there is an increased conversion of 25 (OH) vitamin D to the active form, 1,25 $(OH)_2$ vitamin D.
   j. Familial hypocalcuric hypercalcemia
   k. Lithium. Lithium is thought to increase PTH secretion.
3. Decreased excretion. Thiazide diuretics

Manifestations

The manifestations of hypercalcemia are numerous and non-specific, e.g., "bones, stones, and groans."

HEENT   Corneal calcification ("band" keratopathy)
CVS   Short Q-T interval, prolonged PR interval (Fig. 24–1), dysrhythmias, digoxin sensitivity, hypertension

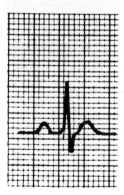

Figure 24–1. Hypercalcemia (short QT interval; prolonged PR interval).

GI	Anorexia, nausea, vomiting, constipation, abdominal pain, pancreatitis ("groans")
GU	Polyuria, polydipsia, nephrolithiasis ("stones")
NEURO	Insomnia, restlessness, delirium, dementia, psychosis, lethargy, coma
MSS	Muscle weakness, hyporeflexia, bone pain, fractures ("bones")
MISC	Hyperchlorhydric metabolic acidosis

Management

Assess the Severity

The severity of the situation should be determined according to the serum calcium concentration, the rate of progression, and the presence or absence of symptoms. It is important to recognize that most laboratories measure total serum calcium (ionized plus albumin bound), but the primary determinant of the physiologic effect is the ionized calcium.

If the patient is hypoalbuminemic, a correction factor can be used to estimate the total calcium concentration. For every 10 gm/L of hypoalbuminemia, add 0.2 mmol/L to the serum calcium value, e.g., if the measured serum calcium value is 2.6 mmol/L (the upper limit of normal) but the serum albumin value is low at 30 gm/L (with an anticipated normal concentration of 40 gm/L), the corrected serum albumin value is 0.2 + 2.6 = 2.8 mmol/L (moderate elevation).

How high is the serum calcium?
Normal range = 2.2 to 2.6 mmol/L
Mild elevation = 2.6 to 2.9 mmol/L
Moderation elevation = 2.9 to 3.2 mmol/L
Severe elevation = >3.2 mmol/L

Is there a continuing cause that is likely to result in further increases?

If the situation is progressive, the patient requires immediate treatment.

Is the patient symptomatic?

Any symptomatic patient requires immediate treatment.

Severe hypercalcemia (>3.2 mmol/L) requires immediate treatment because of the danger of a fatal cardiac dysrhythmia.

1. *Correct volume depletion/expand extracellular volume.* Give NS IV 500 ml as fast as possible. Further NS boluses can be given, dependent on the volume status. Titrate the NS IV maintenance rate to keep the patient slightly volume expanded. If the patient has a history of CHF, this volume expansion should be undertaken in the ICU/CCU since close monitoring of the volume status will be required. A reduction in the serum calcium level will be expected because of hemodilution and because an increased urinary sodium excretion is accompanied by an increased calcium excretion.
2. *Establish diuresis >2500 ml/day.* In addition to maintaining volume expansion with NS, give *furosemide* (Lasix) 20 to 40 mg IV q2 to 4h in order to establish a diuresis of >2500 ml/day. Care must be taken not to induce volume depletion with administration of furosemide. The patient may require 4 to 10 L of NS/day to maintain the volume expanded state. Furosemide inhibits the tubular reabsorption of calcium, thus increasing calcium excretion by the kidneys. Do not use thiazides to establish diuresis since they elevate the serum calcium level.
3. *Dialysis.* Occasionally, when the serum calcium level is extremely high, e.g., >4.5 mmol/L, hemodialysis or peritoneal dialysis may be required.

If *hypercalcemia* is *secondary to neoplasm*, in addition to the administration of NS and furosemide (as previously discussed), one of the following medications may be of value:

1. Corticosteroids: *Prednisone* 5 to 15 mg PO daily or *hydrocortisone* (Solu-Cortef) 40 to 60 mg IV daily in divided doses. Steroids antagonize the peripheral action of vitamin D (decreased absorption, decreased bone mobilization, and decreased renal tubular reabsorption of calcium).
2. *Indomethacin* 50 mg PO q8h. Indomethacin inhibits the synthesis of prostaglandin E_2, which is produced by some solid tumors, e.g., of the breast.
3. *Mithramycin* 15 to 25 mcg/kg in 1 L of NS IV over 3 to 6 hours. Mithramycin inhibits bone resorption. The onset of action is 48 hours.

4. Additional methods of lowering the serum calcium level are available, including calcitonin and diphosphates, but they are associated with major risks and are best avoided.

Moderate hypercalcemia or mild symptomatic hypercalcemia (2.9 to 3.2 mmol/L or lesser elevations in the presence of symptoms).

1. *Correct volume depletion* and expand extracellular fluid volume with NS 500 ml IV given over 1 to 2 hours. Further NS can be given at a rate to keep the patient slightly volume expanded.
2. *Establish diuresis >2500 ml/day* if volume expansion alone is unsuccessful in lowering the serum calcium.
3. *Mild asymptomatic hypercalcemia* (2.6 to 2.9 mmol/L). Mild asymptomatic hypercalcemia does not require immediate treatment. The appropriate investigations may be ordered in the morning.

HYPOCALCEMIA

Causes

1. *Decreased intake/absorption*
   a. Malabsorption
   b. Intestinal bypass surgery
   c. Short bowel syndrome
   d. Vitamin D deficiency
2. *Decreased production/mobilization from bone*
   a. Hypoparathyroidism (following sub-total thyroidectomy or parathyroidectomy)
   b. Pseudohypoparathyroidism
   c. Vitamin D deficiency (decreased production of 25(OH) vitamin D or $1,25(OH)_2$ vitamin D)
   d. Hyperphosphatemia
   e. Acute pancreatitis
   f. Hypomagnesemia
   g. Alkalosis (hyperventilation, vomiting, fistulae)
   h. Neoplasm
      (1) Paradoxical hypocalcemia associated with osteoblastic metastasis (lung, breast, prostate)
      (2) Medullary carcinoma of the thyroid (calcitonin-producing tumor)
      (3) Rapid tumor lysis with phosphate release
3. *Increased excretion*
   a. Chronic renal failure
   b. Loop diuresis
   c. Aminoglycosides

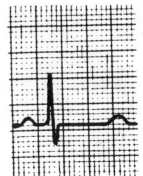

Figure 24–2. Hypocalcemia (long QT interval).

Manifestations

The earliest symptoms are paresthesias of the lips, fingers, and toes.

HEENT   Papilledema, diplopia
CVS   Prolonged QT interval without U-waves (Fig. 24–2)
GI   Abdominal cramps
NEURO   Confusion, irritability, depression
   Hyperactive tendon reflexes
   Carpopedal spasm, laryngospasm (stridor), tetany
   Grand mal seizures
   Paresthesias of lips, fingers, and toes
   Special tests:
   Chvostek's sign (Fig. 24–3)
      Facial muscle spasm elicited by tapping the facial nerve immediately anterior to the ear lobe and below the zygomatic arch. (This is a normal finding in 10% of the population.)
   Trousseau's sign (Fig. 24–4)
      Carpal spasm elicited by occluding the arterial blood flow to the forearm for 3 to 5 minutes.

Management

Assess the Severity

The severity of the situation should be determined according to the serum calcium and phosphate concentrations and the presence or absence of symptoms. If the serum albumin is not within the normal range, a correction factor can be used to estimate the total serum calcium (ionized plus albumin bound). See page 244 for a discussion of this correction factor.

How low is the serum calcium level?

Normal range = 2.2 to 2.6 mmol/L

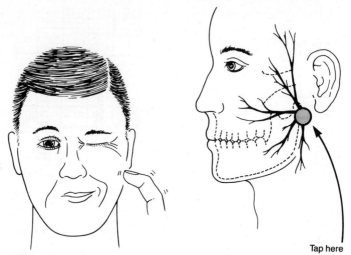

Figure 24–3. Chvostek's sign. Facial muscle spasm elicited by tapping the facial nerve immediately anterior to the earlobe and below the zygomatic arch.

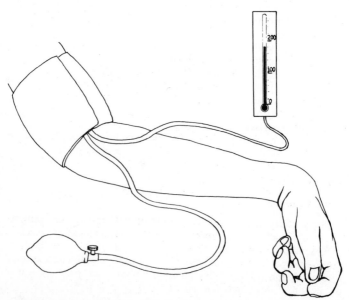

Figure 24–4. Trousseau's sign. Carpal spasm elicited by occluding the arterial blood flow to the forearm for 3 to 5 min.

Mild depletion = 1.9 to 2.2 mmol/L
Moderate depletion = 1.5 to 1.9 mmol/L
Severe depletion = <1.5 mmol/L

What is the serum phosphate concentration?

If the serum phosphate concentration is markedly elevated (>6 mmol/L) in severe hypocalcemia, correction of hyperphosphatemia must be carried out with IV glucose and insulin before calcium is given to avoid metastatic calcification.

Is the patient symptomatic?

Hypocalcemic patients who are asymptomatic do not require urgent correction with IV calcium.

Is the patient receiving digoxin?

Caution is required if the patient is receiving digoxin, since calcium potentiates the action of digoxin. Ideally, if IV calcium administration is required, the patient should have continuous ECG monitoring.

Severe, symptomatic hypocalcemia (<1.5 mmol/L) requires immediate treatment because of the danger of respiratory failure from laryngospasm.

1. Provided the patient's PO_4 is normal or low, give 10 to 20 ml (1 to 2 gm) of 10% solution of calcium gluconate IV in 100 ml D5W over 30 minutes. If the patient has evidence of tetany or laryngeal stridor, the same dose should be given over 2 minutes as a direct injection, i.e., calcium gluconate 10% solution 10 to 20 ml IV over 2 minutes. Oral calcium may be started immediately: 200 mg of elemental calcium q2h × 4 doses. If the corrected serum calcium value is <1.9 mmol/L 6 hours after initiating this treatment, a calcium infusion is required. Add 10 ml (1 gm) of a 10% calcium gluconate solution to 500 ml D5W and infuse over 6 hours. If the serum calcium value is not within the normal range after 6 hours of this infusion, 5 ml (500 mg) of calcium gluconate can be added to the initial infusion dose q6h until a satisfactory serum calcium level is achieved. The post-parathyroidectomy patient may require 1 to 1.5 gm calcium gluconate/hr. Add 100 ml (10 gm) of a 10% calcium gluconate solution to 500 ml D5W and begin the infusion at 50 ml/hr (1 gm/hr).

2. If the patient is hyperphosphatemic (PO_4 >6 mmol/L), correction with glucose and insulin is required prior to administration of IV calcium. Consult the nephrology service immediately.

Mild and moderate, asymptomatic hypocalcemia does not require urgent IV calcium replacement. Oral calcium replacement with elemental calcium 1000 to 1500 mg/day may be started to achieve a corrected serum calcium level in the 2.2 to 2.6 mmol/L range. Long-term treatment with oral calcium or vitamin D depends on the etiology, which can be evaluated in the morning.

25

COAGULATION DISORDERS

SCREENING

The hemostatic system consists of three components that are required to produce a clot as follows: (1) intact *blood vessels* ("vascular factors"), (2) intact *coagulation factors*, and (3) normal, in both number and function, *platelets*. A patient suspected of having a bleeding disorder can be screened by a few routine tests designed to assess the integrity of the hemostatic system.

1. *Activated partial thromboplastin time (aPTT)*. The aPTT tests the intrinsic and common coagulation pathways (factors XII, XI, IX, VIII, X, V, and II) (Fig. 25–1). Occasionally the presence of an "acquired anticoagulant," such as the lupus anticoagulant, will prolong the aPTT. This situation can be differentiated from a factor deficiency by demonstrating failure to normalize the aPTT when a sample of the patient's plasma is mixed with normal plasma 50:50.
2. *Prothrombin time (PT)*. This tests the extrinsic and common coagulation pathways (factors II, V, VII, and X).
3. *Platelet count* tests platelet number.
4. *Bleeding time* tests platelet function and vascular integrity.

These four measurements are screening tests only and will not detect all hemostatic defects. If there is a strong suspicion of an underlying bleeding disorder despite normal hemostatic screening test results one should consider factor XIII deficiency, von Willebrand's disease, or mild hemophilia A or B. Laboratory features of the common coagulation disorders are listed in Table 25–1.

CAUSES

1. *Vessel abnormalities* (vascular factor)
   a. *Hereditary disorders*
      (1) Hereditary hemorrhagic telangiectasia
      (2) Ehlers-Danlos syndrome
      (3) Marfan's syndrome
      (4) Pseudoxanthoma elasticum
      (5) Osteogenesis imperfecta
   b. *Acquired disorders*
      (1) *Vasculitis*
         (a) Schönlein-Henoch purpura
         (b) Systemic lupus erythematosus

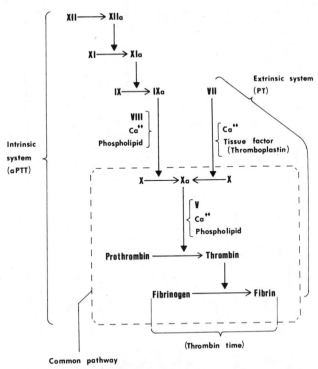

Figure 25–1. The coagulation cascade.

- (c) Polyarteritis nodosa
- (d) Rheumatoid arthritis
- (e) Cryoglobulinemia
- (2) *Increased vascular fragility*
  - (a) Senile purpura
  - (b) Cushing's syndrome
  - (c) Scurvy
2. *Coagulation factor abnormalities* (see Fig. 25–1)
   a. *Congenital*
      (1) Factor VIII deficiency (hemophilia A)
      (2) Factor IX deficiency (hemophilia B)
   b. *Acquired*
      (1) Liver disease
      (2) Vitamin K deficiency
         (a) Inadequate oral intake (e.g., prolonged post-operative course, ICU setting)
         (b) Antibiotic treatment (especially with cephalosporins)
         (c) Malabsorption/steatorrhea
         (d) Liver disease
         (e) Aspirin overdose

Table 25-1. LABORATORY FEATURES OF COMMON COAGULATION DISORDERS

Disorder	Diagnostic Laboratory Tests				
	aPTT	PT	Platelets	Bleeding Time	Other
Vessel Abnormalities					
Vasculitis	Normal	Normal	Normal	Normal or ↑	↑ C3 C4 ↑ C1Q binding
Increased vascular fragility	Normal	Normal	Normal	↑	
Hereditary connective tissue disorders	Normal	Normal	Normal	↑	
Paraproteinemias	Normal	Normal	Normal	↑	
Coagulation Factor Abnormalities					
Heparin	Normal or ↑	↑ or Normal	Normal or →	Normal or ↑	
Warfarin	↑	↑	Normal	Normal	
Vitamin K deficiency	↑	↑	Normal	Normal	
DIC	↑	↑	→	Normal or ↑*	↑ Fibrin degradation products; ↓ fibrinogen
Factor VIII deficiency	↑	Normal	Normal	Normal	↓ Factor VIII assay
Factor IX deficiency	↑	Normal	Normal	Normal	Normal Factor IX assay
Von Willebrand's disease	Normal or ↑	Normal	Normal or →	Normal or ↑	Normal or ↓ Factor VIII assay Normal or ↓ Factor VIII antigen ↓ Ristocetin cofactor
Liver disease	↑	↑	Normal or →	Normal or ↑	
Platelet Disorders					
Thrombocytopenia	Normal	Normal	→	↑	
Impaired platelet function	Normal	Normal	Normal	Normal or ↑*	

*Depends on degree of thrombocytopenia.

- (3) Disseminated intravascular coagulation
    - (a) Infection (e.g., gram-negative sepsis)
    - (b) Obstetric catastrophes
    - (c) Malignancy (e.g., prostatic cancer)
    - (d) Tissue damage/shock
- (4) Anticoagulants/thrombolytics
    - (a) Heparin
    - (b) Warfarin
    - (c) Streptokinase
    - (d) Tissue plasminogen activator
- (5) Massive transfusion (depletion of factors V and VIII)
- (6) Circulating anticoagulants, e.g., lupus anticoagulant or factor specific anticoagulants

3. *Platelet abnormalities*
    a. Thrombocytopenia
    - (1) *Decreased marrow production*
      Marrow replacement by tumor, granuloma (e.g., TB, sarcoid), fibrous tissue
      Storage diseases (e.g., Gaucher's disease)
      Marrow injury by drugs (e.g., sulfonamides, chloramphenicol)
      Defecefective maturation (e.g., B_{12} or folate deficiency)
    - (2) *Increased peripheral destruction*
        - (a) Immune mediated
            - i. Drugs (e.g., quinine/quinidine, heparin)
            - ii. Connective tissue disorders (e.g., systemic lupus erythematosus)
            - iii. Lymphoproliferative disorders (e.g., CLL)
            - iv. Idiopathic
            - v. Post-transfusion purpura
        - (b) Non-immune mediated
            - i. Consumption (e.g., DIC, TTP, prosthetic valves)
            - ii. Dilutional (e.g., massive transfusion)
        - (c) Sequestration (e.g., any cause of splenomegaly)
    b. Impaired platelet function
    - (1) *Hereditary*
        - (a) Von Willebrand's disease
        - (b) Bernard-Soulier disease
        - (c) Glanzmann's thromboasthenia
    - (2) *Acquired*
        - (a) Drugs (e.g., NSAIDs; aspirin; antibiotics, such as high-dose penicillin, cephalosporins, nitrofurantoin)
        - (b) Uremia
        - (c) Paraproteins (e.g., amyloidosis, multiple myeloma, Waldenström's macroglobulinema)
        - (d) Myeloproliferative diseases (e.g., CGL, essential thrombocytosis)

MANIFESTATIONS

Bleeding in the patient with a coagulation disorder is of concern for two reasons as follows:

1. Progressive loss of intravascular volume, if uncorrected, may lead to hypovolemic shock with inadequate perfusion of vital organs.
2. Hemorrhage into specific organ sites may produce local tissue or organ injury (e.g., intracerebral hemorrhage, epidural hemorrhage with spinal cord compression, hemarthrosis)

Though "bleeding" is the clinical manifestation that alerts one to the possibility of a coagulation disorder, the three types of disorders (vessel abnormalities, coagulation factor deficiencies, and platelet abnormalities) are said to have different clinical presentations.

Patients with *vessel or platelet abnormalities* who are bleeding may present with petechiae, purpura, or easy bruisability. The bleeding characteristically occurs superficially (e.g., oozing from mucous membranes or IV sites). The bleeding of scurvy is seen only rarely in North America and is usually manifested by perifollicular hemorrhages, though gingival bleeding and intramuscular hematomas may also occur.

Bleeding due to *coagulation factor deficiencies* may occur spontaneously, in deeper organ sites, e.g., visceral hemorrhages, hemarthroses, and tends to be delayed and prolonged. Bleeding associated with thrombolytic agents is usually manifested by continuous oozing from IV sites.

MANAGEMENT

1. *Vessel abnormalities*. Treatment of bleeding due to vessel abnormalities is usually treatment of the underlying disorder.
   a. Serious bleeding due to *hereditary disorders of connective tissue* and to hereditary hemorrhagic telangiectasia most often requires local mechanical or surgical measures at the site of hemorrhage in order to control blood loss.
   b. In the *vasculitides*, control of bleeding is best achieved by use of corticosteroids, other immunosuppressive agents, or a combination of both.
   c. There is no good treatment for the increased vascular fragility that results in *senile purpura*. Purpura due to *Cushing's syndrome* is preventable with normalization of plasma cortisol levels. However, in the patient receiving therapeutic corticosteroids, the underlying indication for therapy often prevents significant reduction of steroid levels. Hemorrhages associated with *scurvy* will not recur following adequate dietary supplementation of ascorbic acid.

2. *Coagulation factor abnormalities.* Treatment of coagulation factor abnormalities is dependent upon the specific factor deficiency or deficiencies.

   a. *Specific factor deficiencies* should always be treated in consultation with a hematologist. Factor VIII deficiency (hemophilia A) can be treated with Factor VIII concentrate or cryoprecipitate. Non-blood products may also be of benefit, e.g., DDAVP, danazole. Factor IX deficiency (hemophilia B) may be treated with Factor IX concentrate or banked plasma.

   b. *Liver disease.* Because patients with liver disease are frequently also vitamin K–deficient, it is worthwhile to administer *vitamin K* 10 mg SC or IV daily for 3 days. IV vitamin K has occasionally caused anaphylactic reactions. If the patient does not respond to vitamin K, bleeding should be managed by transfusion of fresh frozen plasma. Factor IX concentrates carry a risk of thromboembolism and are contraindicated in liver disease.

   c. *Vitamin K deficiency* may be treated in an identical manner to that subsequently outlined for correction of warfarin coagulopathy. Ideally, however, one should identify and treat the underlying cause of vitamin K deficiency.

   d. The treatment of *DIC* is both complicated and controversial. All medical authorities agree, however, that definitive management involves treating the underlying cause. Additionally, a patient with DIC often requires coagulation factor and platelet support in the form of fresh frozen plasma, cryoprecipitate, and platelet transfusions. The role of heparin in the treatment of DIC is controversial and should not be instituted prior to hematologic consultation.

   e. Bleeding due to *anticoagulant therapy* can be reversed slowly or rapidly depending upon the clinical status of the patient and the site of bleeding. Heparin has a half-life of only 1½ hours, and simply discontinuing a heparin infusion should normalize the aPTT and correct the heparin-induced coagulapathy in minor episodes of bleeding. Serious bleeding complications can be treated by discontinuing the heparin infusion and reversing the heparin effect with *protamine sulfate* 1 mg/100 units of heparin (approximately) IV slowly. Dosage is determined by estimating the amount of circulating heparin and should be limited to no more than 50 mg per single dose in a 10 minute period. Side effects of protamine include hypotension, bradycardia, flushing, and bleeding.

   Rapid reversal of warfarin effect, as may be required in life-threatening hemorrhages, can be achieved by administering *plasma* (e.g., 2 units at a time) with subsequent redetermination of PT. Although both fresh frozen plasma and banked plasma contain the vitamin K–dependent clotting factors, banked plasma is considerably less expensive and hence is the replacement solution of choice. Severe bleeding (e.g., intracranial hemorrhage) requires urgent hematologic consultation. When prolonged reversal of anticoagulant effect is desired, *vitamin K* 10 mg PO, SC, or IV may be given daily for 3 days. Minor bleeding complications in patients on warfarin may require temporary discontinuation of this drug. IV vitamin K has occasionally caused anaphylactic reaction and hence should be given with caution.

f. *Bleeding due to thrombolytic agents.* Localized oozing at sites of invasive procedures often can be controlled by local pressure dressings or avoided in the first place by not doing invasive procedures. More serious hemorrhage requires discontinuation of the thrombolytic agent. Fibrinolytic agents that are not fibrin specific will cause systemic fibrinogenolysis, and therefore fresh frozen plasma may be required to replace fibrinogen. *Aminocaproic acid*, which is an inhibitor of plasminogen activator, has also been used (20 to 30 gm/day) but should not be initiated prior to hematologic consultation.

3. *Platelet abnormalities.* Treatment of bleeding in the thrombocytopenic patient varies depending on the presence of either an abnormality in platelet production or an increase in platelet destruction.

a. *Decreased marrow production* of platelets is treated in the long term by identifying and, if possible, correcting the underlying cause (e.g., chemotherapy for tumor, removal of marrow toxins, B_{12} or folate supplementation when indicated). In the short term, however, a serious bleeding complication should be treated by platelet transfusion (e.g., 6 to 8 units at a time). One unit of platelets can be expected to increase the platelet count by 1000 in the patient with inadequate marrow production of platelets. Check the response to transfusion by ordering a 1 hour post-platelet transfusion count.

b. *Increased peripheral destruction* of platelets is also best managed by identifying and correcting the underlying problem. Often this management involves the systemic use of corticosteroids or other immunosuppressive agents. The patient tends to have less serious bleeding manifestations than one with inadequate marrow production of platelets but may require platelet transfusion for life-threatening bleeding episodes. There are exceptions to platelet transfusion therapy in thrombocytopenia in the patient with thrombotic thrombocytopenic purpura—in this situation platelet transfusions should be avoided since they may actually worsen the condition.

c. *Dilutional thrombocytopenia* due to massive RBC transfusion and IV fluid therapy is treated with platelet transfusion as required. Dilutional thrombocytopenia can usually be prevented by remembering to transfuse 8 units of platelets for every 10 to 12 units of RBCs transfused.

d. *Von Willebrand's disease* may be treated with cryoprecipitate or DDAVP.

e. *Bleeding disorders resulting from acquired platelet dysfunction* are best managed by identification and correction of the underlying problem. Temporary treatment of bleeding disorders due to these conditions may involve platelet transfusion or other more specialized measures (e.g., cryoprecipitate, DDAVP, conjugated estrogens in uremia).

HYPERGLYCEMIA

Causes

Patients with Documented Diabetes Mellitus

- Poorly controlled IDDM or NIDDM
- Stress (surgery, infection, severe illness)
- Drugs (corticosteroids, thiazides)
- TPN administration

Patients without Previously Documented Diabetes Mellitus

- New onset of diabetes mellitus
- TPN administration
- Drugs (corticosteroids, thiazides)

Acute Manifestations

Mild Hyperglycemia (Fasting Blood Glucose of 6.1 to 11.0 mmol/L)

- Polyuria, polydipsia, thirst

Moderate Hyperglycemia (Fasting Blood Glucose of 11.1 to 22.5 mmol/L)

- Decreased JVP (volume depletion)
- Polyuria, polydipsia, thirst

Severe Hyperglycemia (Fasting Blood Glucose of > 22.5 mol/L)
IDDM

- Musty odor on breath (ketone breath)
- Kussmaul's breathing (deep, pauseless respirations seen when pH is < 7.2)
- Decreased JVP (volume depletion)
- Anorexia, nausea, vomiting, abdominal pain (may mimic a "surgical abdomen")
- Ileus, gastric dilatation
- Hyporeflexia, hypotonia, delirium, coma

NIDDM

- Polyuria, polydipsia
- Volume depletion
- Confusion, coma

Management

Assess the Severity

The severity of the situation should be determined according to the blood glucose level and the patient's symptoms.

	Fasting or AC Blood Glucose (mmol/L)	Two-hour PC Blood Glucose (mmol/L)
Normal range	3.5–6.0	<11.0
Mild hyperglycemia	6.1–11.0	11.1–16.5
Moderate hyperglycemia	11.1–22.5	16.6–27.5
Severe hyperglycemia	>22.5	>27.5

Mild, asymptomatic hyperglycemia does not require urgent treatment. Order the following:

1. Fasting blood glucose in the morning.
   A fasting blood glucose of > 7.8 mmol/L on more than one occasion confirms the diagnosis of diabetes mellitus. Make sure the patient is not receiving glucose-containing IV solutions that will make these results invalid. In addition, the diagnosis of diabetes mellitus cannot be made in the setting of stress (e.g., infection, surgery, severe illness). The criterion for the diagnosis of diabetes mellitus is as follows:

   Fasting blood glucose > 7.8 mmol/L $\times$ 2
   or
   Random blood sugar > 11.1 mmol/L $\times$ 2
   or
   A GTT with fasting blood glucose < 7.8 mmol/L and a 2-hour PC > 11.1 mmol/L.
2. Chemstrip or Glucometer readings AC meals and QHS.
   If the readings are > 25 or < 2.8 mmol/L, a stat blood glucose sample should be drawn and a physician informed.
   Moderate hyperglycemia may require an adjustment of the insulin being given. Examine the diabetic record for the past 3 days.
   A sample adjustment in dosage is subsequently tabulated. The Chemstrip or Glucometer readings are in mmol/L; the SC insulin dose given is indicated in parentheses (e.g., 20/10 indicates that 20 units of NPH and 10 units of regular insulin have been given.)

	AC Breakfast NPH/REG	AC Lunch NPH/REG	AC Supper NPH/REG	QHS NPS/REG
Aug. 1	16.7 (20/10)	13.9 (0/0)	16.7 (10/10)	18.1 (0/0)
Aug. 2	13.9 (20/10)	16.7 (0/4)	8.3 (10/10)	19.4 (0/0)
Aug. 3	16.7 (20/10)	15.2 (0/0)	113.1 (10/10)	25.0 (0/0)

You have been called at night on August 3rd because of the Chemstrip or Glucometer reading of 25.0 mmol/L. Order the following:

1. Stat random blood glucose to confirm the Chemstrip or Glucometer reading.
2. Regular insulin 5 to 10 units SC now. The main consideration now is not to devise a schedule that will achieve perfect blood glucose control for the remainder of the patient's hospital stay— short-term control of blood glucose levels has not been shown to decrease cardiovascular complications in the diabetic. When the blood glucose level is elevated at night your aim is to prevent the development of ketoacidosis in the patient with IDDM or of the hyperosmolar state in the patient with NIDDM without producing symptomatic hypoglycemia with your treatment.
3. Determining the reason for poor control of blood glucose AC breakfast may aid in an ongoing adjustment of the patient's insulin. This can be achieved by ordering an 0300H Chemstrip or a Glucometer reading. Hypoglycemia documented at 0300H would suggest that AC breakfast hyperglycemia is due to hyperglycemic rebound (the Somogyi effect), which is correctly managed by reducing the AC supper NPH insulin dose. Hyperglycemia documented at 0300H would suggest that AC breakfast hyperglycemia is due to inadequate insulin coverage overnight; this is correctly managed by increasing the AC supper NPH insulin dose.

Severe hyperglycemia requires urgent treatment.

1. *IDDM—Diabetic Ketoacidosis.* This complication may be seen in the patient with poorly controlled IDDM. It is due to an absolute insulin deficit resulting in impaired resynthesis of long-chain fatty acids from acetate, with subsequent conversion to the acidic ketone bodies (ketosis).
   a. *Correct volume depletion.* Give 500 ml NS IV as fast as possible, with further IV rates guided by reassessment of volume status. If the patient has a history of CHF, weight < 50 kg, or is ≥ 80 years of age, NS should be given cautiously, to avoid iatrogenic CHF.
   b. *Begin an insulin infusion.* Give 5 to 10 units of IV regular insulin as a single dose by direct slow injection followed by an infusion rate based on close monitoring of Chemstrip or Glucometer readings; initially, hourly measurements may be required. Regular insulin can bind to the plastic IV tubing. In order to ensure accurate insulin delivery, 30 to 50 ml of of the infusion solution should be run through the IV tubing and discarded, before connecting the IV tubing to the patient. Discontinue the standing order for SC insulin or oral hypoglycemics, prior to beginning the insulin infusion. Start the insulin infusion at 0.1 U/kg/hr until the plasma

glucose reaches 14 mmol/L and then discontinue the insulin infusion and begin an IV of D5W. Expect the plasma glucose level to fall 20 mmol/L/hour. If this is not achieved, the patient has insulin resistance, and the insulin infusion rate will need to be increased to 0.15 to 0.2 U/kg/hr.

   c. *Monitor blood glucose, serum electrolytes, and ABGs.* Hyperglycemic patients can have metabolic acidemia and hypokalemia. As NS and insulin are administered, the acidemia is corrected, and the potassium shifts into the cells from the extracellular fluid; this can result in worsening of the hypokalemia. Order baseline ABGs, electrolytes, urea, creatinine, and glucose levels. Repeat the ABGs and potassium level in 2 hours and thereafter as required. When hypokalemia is first noted, add KCl to the IV NS, provided the patient is passing urine and has normal urea and creatinine levels. If the patient is in renal failure, caution should be taken in adding any potassium to the IV, in order to avoid iatrogenic hyperkalemia.

   d. *Search for the precipitating cause.* Common precipitating factors include the following:
      (1) Infection
      (2) Inadequate insulin dosage
      (3) Dietary indiscretion
      (4) Pancreatitis

2. *NIDDM—Hyperosmolar, Hyperglycemic, Non-Ketotic State.* This condition may be seen in a patient with poorly controlled NIDDM. Typically, the patient is 50 to 70 years old; many will present without prior histories of diabetes mellitus. The precipitating event is often stroke, infection, pancreatitis, or drugs. The blood glucose level is often very high (e.g., > 55 mmol/L), but ketosis is absent.

   a. *Correct volume depletion and water deficit.* The objective of fluid therapy in the non-ketotic hyperosmolar state is to both correct the volume deficit and resolve the hyperosmolarity. These can be achieved by giving 500 ml of NS IV over 2 hours, with further IV rates guided by reassessment of volume status. Once the volume deficit is corrected using NS, remaining water deficits, as indicated by persistent hypernatremia or hyperglycemia, are best corrected using hypotonic IV solutions, such as 1/2 NS.

   b. *Begin an insulin infusion.* See previous discussion of treatment of diabetic ketoacidosis.

   c. *Monitor blood glucose level and serum electrolytes.* Order baseline electrolytes, urea, creatinine, and glucose levels. Repeat the blood glucose level and electrolytes in 2 hours and thereafter as required.

   d. *Search for the precipitating cause.*
      (1) Infection

(2) Inadequate fluid intake
(3) Other acute illnesses (MI, stroke)

HYPOGLYCEMIA

Causes

Patients with Documented Diabetes Mellitus

- Excess insulin or oral hypoglycemic administration
- Decreased caloric intake
- Missed meals or missed snacks
- Increased exercise

Patients without Documented Diabetes Mellitus

- Surreptitious intake of insulin or oral hypoglycemics
- Insulinoma
- Supervised 72-hour fasting for the investigation of hypoglycemia
- Drugs (ethanol, pentamidine, disopyramide, MAO inhibitors)
- Hepatic failure
- Adrenal insufficiency

Manifestations

Adrenergic Response (i.e., Catecholamine Release due to a Rapid Decrease in Glucose Level). Diaphoresis, palpitations, tremulousness, tachycardia, hunger, acral and perioral numbness, anxiety, combativeness, confusion, coma.

CNS Response (Slow Response May Develop Over 1 to 3 Days). Headaches, diplopia, bizarre behavior, focal neurologic deficits, confusion, seizures, and coma.

Patients receiving oral hypoglycemics may not experience the adrenergic response and develop confusion and coma unrecognized as hypoglycemia.

Management

Assess the Severity

Any symptomatic patient with suspected hypoglycemia requires treatment. Symptoms can be precipitated by either a rapid fall in blood glucose level or an absolute low level of blood glucose.

1. *Draw 1 ml of blood* to be sent for blood glucose testing to confirm the diagnosis. If the cause of hypoglycemia is not clear, draw 10 ml, and ask the laboratory to save an aliquot for possible later insulin and C peptide measurement. Insulin produced endogenously includes the C peptide fragment, in contrast

to commercial preparations of insulin. A high insulin level associated with a high C peptide fragment and hypoglycemia suggests endogenous production of excess insulin (e.g., insulinoma), whereas a high insulin level associated with a low C peptide level and hypoglycemia suggests surreptitious or therapeutic administration of exogenous insulin.

2. In the cooperative awake patient oral glucose in the form of sweetened fruit juice may be given. If the patient is unable to take oral fluids or is unconscious D50W 50 ml IV should be given by direct, slow injection. If there is no IV access and the patient is unable to take oral fluids (e.g., unconscious), *glucagon* 0.5 to 1.0 mg SC or IM should be given.

3. If ongoing hypoglycemia is anticipated or if the patient's symptoms were severe (e.g., seizure, coma), begin a maintenance IV of D5W or D10W at a rate of 100 ml/hr. Ask the RN to reassess the patient in 1 hour. In addition, remeasure the blood glucose level in 2 to 4 hours to ensure that hypoglycemic relapse has not occurred. Hypoglycemia due to oral hypoglycemics may require repeated doses of D50W because of the slow metabolism and excretion of these drugs.

27

POTASSIUM DISORDERS

HYPERKALEMIA

Causes

Excessive Intake

- Potassium supplements (PO or IV)
- "Salt substitutes"
- High-dose IV therapy with potassium salts of penicillin
- Blood transfusions

Decreased Excretion

- Renal failure (acute or chronic)
- Potassium-sparing diuretics (spironolactone, triamterene, amiloride)
- Addison's disease, hypoaldosteronism
- Distal tubular dysfunction (i.e., type IV RTA)

Shift from Intracellular to Extracellular Fluid

- Acidemia (especially non-anion gap)
- Insulin deficiency
- Tissue destruction (hemolysis, crush injuries, rhabdomyolysis)
- Drugs (succinylcholine, digoxin, arginine, beta blockers)
- Hyperkalemic periodic paralysis

Factitious

- Prolonged tourniquet placement for venipuncture
- Blood sample hemolysis
- Leukocytosis
- Thrombocytosis

Manifestations

Cardiac

- Fatal ventricular dysrhythmias

The progressive ECG changes seen in hyperkalemia are peaked T waves → depressed ST segments → decreased amplitude of R waves → prolonged PR interval → small or absent P waves → wide QRS complexes → sine wave pattern (Fig. 27–1).

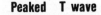

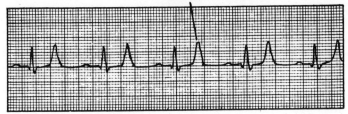

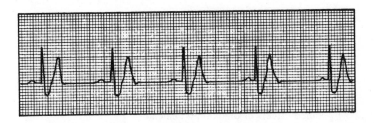

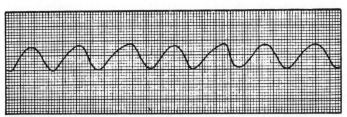

Figure 27–1. Progressive electrocardiographic manifestations of hyperkalemia.

Neuromuscular

- Weakness
- Paresthesias
- Depressed deep tendon reflexes

Management

ECG

Fatal ventricular dysrhythmias can occur at any time during treatment, and hence continuous ECG monitoring is required if the potassium level is above 6.5 mmol/L.

Assess the Severity

The severity of the situation should be determined according to the serum potassium concentration, the ECG findings, and whether or not the underlying cause is immediately remediable.

If *severe*

- Serum $K^+ > 8.0$ mmol/L
- ECG findings more advanced than peaked T waves alone
- Cause not immediately remediable

1. Notify your resident.
2. Place the patient on continuous ECG monitoring.
3. Correct contributing factors (acidemia, hypovolemia).
4. Give one or more of the following:
   a. *Calcium gluconate*: 5 to 10 ml of a 10% solution given IV over 2 minutes. This will temporarily antagonize the cardiac and neuromuscular effects of hyperkalemia. Calcium gluconate's onset is immediate, and its effect lasts 1 hour. It will not, however, reduce the serum concentration of potassium. *Caution*: Administration of calcium to the patient on digoxin may precipitate ventricular dysrhythmias due to the combined effects of digoxin and calcium.
   b. *D50W*: 50 ml IV followed by *regular insulin* 5 to 10 units IV will shift potassium from the ECF to the ICF; its effect is immediate and lasts 1 to 2 hours.
   c. *Sodium bicarbonate*: 1 amp (44.6 mmol) IV will shift potassium from the ECF to the ICF; its effect is immediate and lasts 1 to 2 hours.
   d. Give a *glucose-insulin-HCO₃ "cocktail"*: D10W 1000 ml with three ampules of $NaHCO_3$ and 20 units of regular insulin at 75 ml/hr until more definite measures are taken.
   e. *Sodium polystyrene sulfonate* (Kayexalate): 15 to 30 gm (4 to 8 teaspoonfuls) in 50 to 100 ml of 20% sorbitol PO q3 to 4h or 50 gm in 200 ml 20% sorbitol or D20W PR by retention enema for 30 to 60 minutes q4h. This is the only drug treatment that will actually remove potassium from the total body pool.
5. *Hemodialysis* should be considered on an urgent basis if the aforementioned measures have failed or if the patient is in acute or chronic oliguric renal failure. *Peritoneal dialysis* may be preferable in the patient who is hemodynamically unstable.
6. Monitor the serum potassium concentration every 1 to 2 hours until it is below 6.5 mmol/L.

If *moderate*

- Serum K^+ between 6.5 and 8.0 mmol/L
- ECG findings show peaked T waves only.
- Cause is not progressive.

1. Place the patient on continuous ECG monitoring.
2. Correct contributing factors (acidemia, hypovolemia).
3. Give one or more of the following in the dosages previously outlined:
   a. $NaHCO_3$
   b. Glucose and insulin
   c. Sodium polystyrene sulfonate
4. Monitor the serum potassium concentration every 1 to 2 hours until it is below 6.5 mmol/L.

If *mild*

- Serum K^+ > 6.5 mmol/L
- ECG findings show peaked T waves only.
- Cause is not progressive.

1. Correct contributing factors (acidemia, hypovolemia).
2. Remeasure the serum potassium concentration 4 to 6 hours later, depending upon the cause.

HYPOKALEMIA

Causes

Renal Losses (Urine K^+ >20 mmol/Day)
- Diuretics, osmotic diuresis
- Antibiotics (carbenicillin, ticarcillin, nafcillin, amphotericin, aminoglycosides)
- RTA (classic type 1)
- Hyperaldosteronism
- Glucocorticoid excess
- Magnesium deficiency
- Chronic metabolic alkalosis
- Bartter's syndrome
- Fanconi's syndrome
- Ureterosigmoidostomy
- Vomiting, NG suction (Hydrogen ions are lost with vomiting and NG suction, inducing alkalosis that results in renal potassium wasting.)

Extrarenal Losses (Urine K^+ < 20 mmol/Day)
- Diarrhea, laxative abuse
- Intestinal fistula

Inadequate Intake
- Over 1 to 2 weeks

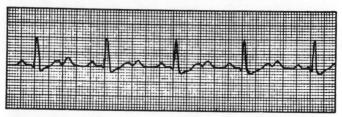

Figure 27–2. Electrocardiographic manifestations of hypokalemia.

Shift from the Extracellular to the Intracellular Space
- Acute alkalosis
- Insulin therapy
- Vitamin B_{12} therapy
- Hypokalemic periodic paralysis
- Salbutamol
- Lithium

Manifestations

Cardiac

- Premature atrial contractions
- Premature ventricular contractions
- Digoxin toxicity
- ECG changes (Fig. 27–2)
  - T-wave flattening
  - U waves
  - ST segment depression

Neuromuscular

- Weakness
- Depressed deep tendon reflexes
- Paresthesias
- Ileus

Miscellaneous

- Nephrogenic diabetes insipidus
- Metabolic alkalosis
- Worsening of hepatic encephalopathy

Management

If possible, correct the underlying cause.

Assess the Severity

The severity of the situation should be determined according to the serum potassium concentration, the ECG findings, and the clinical setting in which hypokalemia is occurring.

If *severe*

■ Serum K^+ < 3.0 mmol/L with PVCs in the setting of myocardial ischemia or with digoxin toxicity.

1. Notify your resident.
2. Place the patient on continuous ECG monitoring.
3. IV replacement therapy may be required, i.e., 10 mmol KCl in 100 ml D5W given IV over 1 hour. Repeat once or twice as necessary. KCl in small volumes should be given through central IV lines, as these high concentrations of potassium are sclerosing to peripheral veins. Further replacement can be achieved with maintenance therapy containing up to 40 to 60 mmol KCl/L of IV fluid at a maximum rate of 20 mmol/hr. Potassium can also be given by the administration of the liquid salt by NG tube or by oral supplementation.
4. Recheck serum potassium concentration after each 20 to 30 mmol IV KCl has been given.

If *moderate*

■ Serum K^+ ≤ 3.0 mmol/L with PACs but no (or infrequent) PVCs and no digoxin toxicity.

1. Notify your resident.
2. Oral potassium supplementation is usually adequate, e.g., Slow-K = 8 mmol KCl per tablet, Kay Ciel Elixir = 20 mmol/15 ml, and K-Lyte = 25 mmol/packet.
3. IV replacement therapy in this situation should be reserved for patients with marked hypokalemia or patients who are unable to take oral supplements (see previous recommendations).
4. Recheck serum potassium concentration in the morning, or sooner if clinically indicated.

If *mild*

■ Serum K^+ between 3.1 and 3.5 mmol/L, no (or infrequent) PVCs, and patient asymptomatic.

1. Oral supplementation is usually adequate (see previous recommendations).
2. Recheck serum potassium concentration in the morning, or sooner if clinically indicated.

REMEMBER

1. Serious hyperkalemia has occurred as a result of potassium supplementation. Hence, serum potassium levels should be

closely monitored during treatment. Be particularly cautious in patients with renal impairment!

2. Hypokalemia and hypocalcemia may coexist. Correction of hypokalemia without accompanying correction of hypocalcemia may increase the risk of ventricular dysrhythmias.

3. Hypokalemia and hypomagnesemia may coexist. Correction of hypokalemia may be unsuccessful unless hypomagnesemia is corrected simultaneously.

28

SODIUM DISORDERS

HYPERNATREMIA
Causes

Inadequate Intake of Water

- Coma
- Hypothalamic dysfunction

Excessive Water Losses

Renal Losses

- Diabetes insipidus
    Nephrogenic
    Pituitary
- Osmotic diuresis
    Hyperglycemia
    Mannitol administration
    Urea

Extrarenal Losses

- Vomiting, NG suction
- Diarrhea
- Sweating (e.g., febrile illnesses)
- Insensible losses (e.g., tachypnea)

Excessive Sodium Gain

- Iatrogenic (excessive sodium administration)
- Primary hyperaldosteronism

Manifestations

Hypernatremia most often results from ECF volume depletion due to hypotonic fluid loss (e.g., vomiting, diarrhea, sweating, osmotic diuresis). Symptoms are dependent on the absolute increase in serum osmolality as well as the rate at which it develops. The manifestations of hypernatremia are due to acute brain cell shrinkage from an outward shift of intracellular water, which occurs as a result of increased ECF osmolality, and range from confusion and muscle irritability to seizures, respiratory paralysis, and death.

Management

1. *Assess the severity.*
   The severity of the situation should be determined according to the symptomatic state of the patient, the serum sodium concentration, the serum osmolality, and the ECF volume.
   a. Osmolality can be measured in the laboratory. However, sufficient information may be available to permit its calculation from knowledge of the major osmotically active substances in the ECF.

   $$\text{Osmolality (mmol/kg)} = \begin{array}{l} 2 \text{ Na (mmol/L)} + \text{urea (mmol/L)} \\ + \text{glucose (mmol/L)} \end{array}$$

   The normal range is 281 to 297 mmol/kg.
   b. Most patients with hypernatremia have an accompanying extracellular volume deficit which can compromise perfusion of vital organs. Assess the volume status of the patient (see Chapter 3).
   c. Most patients with hypernatremia have relatively few symptoms and are not at immediate risk of dying!
2. If possible correct the cause, which is usually evident from the history and physical findings.
3. Correct volume and water deficits. The choice of fluid is dependent on the severity of the extracellular volume deficit.
   a. In patients who are volume depleted, hypernatremia can be corrected by giving IV NS until the patient is hemodynamically stable and then changing to ½ NS or D5W to correct the remaining water deficit.
   b. In patients who are not volume depleted, ½ NS or D5W can be used to correct the water deficit.
   An estimation of the volume of water required can be calculated, remembering that the deficit is in *total body water* which is approximately 60% of body weight.

$$\text{Water deficit} = \frac{\text{Serum Na (observed)} - \text{Serum Na (normal)} \times 0.6 \text{ wt (kg)}}{\text{Serum Na (normal)}}$$

EXAMPLE

A 65-year-old man is admitted to the hospital after being found in his apartment 2 days after falling and fracturing his hip. He is moderately volume depleted and has a serum sodium value of 156 mmol/L. His weight is 70 kg. To calculate the volume of water required to correct the serum sodium:

$$\text{Free water deficit} = \frac{156 \text{ mmol/L} - 140 \text{ mmol/L}}{140 \text{ mmol/L}} \times 0.6(70 \text{ L}) = 4.8 \text{ L}$$

Remember to correct the osmolality abnormality at a rate similar to the rate at which it developed. Biologic systems are more responsive to rates of change than to absolute amounts of change. It is safest to correct half the deficit and then re-evaluate. More rapid corrections than 1 to 2 mmol/L/hr in serum sodium can lead to brain swelling, resulting in the development of confusion seizures, or coma.

   c. In the occasional patient with hypernatremia who is volume *overloaded,* the hypernatremia can be corrected by initiating a diuresis using *furosemide* (Lasix) 20 to 40 mg IV and repeating at intervals of 2 to 4 hours as necessary. Once the extracellular volume has returned to normal, if the serum sodium level is still elevated, then diuresis should be continued, with urinary volume losses replaced with D5W until the serum Na repeats level is again in the normal range.

HYPONATREMIA

Causes

Hyponatremia with Decreased ECF Volume

Renal Loss of Sodium

- Diuretic excess
- Na-losing nephritis
- Diuretic phase of acute tubular necrosis
- Bartter's syndrome
- Hypoaldosteronism

Extrarenal Losses of Sodium

- Vomiting, NG suction
- Diarrhea
- Sweating
- Burns
- Pancreatitis

Hyponatremia with ECF Volume Excess and Edema

- Renal failure
- Nephrotic syndrome
- CHF
- Cirrhosis of the liver

Hyponatremia with Normal Extracellular Fluid Volume

SIADH

Tumors

- Oat cell carcinoma of the lung
- Pancreatic carcinoma
- Duodenal adenocarcinoma

CNS Disorders

- Brain tumors
- Brain trauma
- Meningitis
- Encephalitis

Pulmonary Disorders

- Tuberculosis
- Pneumonia

Drugs

- Chlorpropamide
- Clofibrate
- Cyclophosphamide
- Vincristine
- Carbamazepine
- Narcotics
- Tricyclic antidepressants
- Idiopathic

Pseudohyponatremia

Hyponatremia with Normal Serum Osmolality

- Hyperlipidemia
- Hyperproteinemia

Hyponatremia with Increased Serum Osmolality

- Excess urea
- Hyperglycemia
- Mannitol
- Ethanol
- Methanol
- Ethylene glycol
- Isopropyl alcohol

Endocrine Disorders

- Hypothyroidism
- Addison's disease

Manifestations

Manifestations of hyponatremia depend on the absolute decrease in the serum osmolality, the rate of development of hyponatremia, and the volume status of the patient. When associated with a decreased serum osmolality, hyponatremia may cause the following:

- Confusion
- Lethargy
- Weakness
- Nausea and vomiting
- Seizures
- Coma

When hyponatremia develops gradually, a patient may tolerate a serum sodium concentration of less than 110 mmol/L with only moderate confusion or lethargy. However, a patient in whom the serum sodium concentration decreases rapidly from 140 to 115 mmol/L may present with a seizure.

Management

1. *Assess the severity.* The severity of the situation should be determined according to the symptomatic state of the patient, the serum sodium concentration, the serum osmolality, and the ECF.

   Remember that when attempting to correct disorders manifested by hyponatremia, brain cells attempt to maintain their volume in dilutional states by losing solutes (e.g., potassium). If the serum sodium level is corrected too rapidly (i.e., to levels greater than 120 to 125 mmol/L) the serum may become hypertonic relative to brain cells, resulting in an outward shift of water with resultant CNS damage due to acute brain shinkage.
2. If possible, correct the cause of the hyponatremia. Conditions causing renal losses of sodium are usually accompanied by a urine sodium concentration >20 mmol/L, whereas extrarenal losses of sodium are usually accompanied by an attempt at renal preservation of sodium, i.e., a urine sodium of <10 mmol/L.
3. Assess the volume status of the patient (see Chapter 3).
   a. If the patient is volume depleted correct the ECF volume using NS. Aim for a JVP 2 to 3 cm H_2O above the sternal angle. In this case, the amount of sodium required to improve the serum sodium concentration can be calculated using the following formula:

      mmol Na = Serum Na (desired) − Serum Na (observed) × TBW
      (where TBW = 0.6 × wt in kg)

Remember that biologic systems are more responsive to rates of change than to absolute amounts of change. Make corrections at a rate similar to the rate at which the abnormality developed. It is safest to correct half the deficit and reassess the situation.

EXAMPLE

For a 70-kg man in whom you want to raise the serum sodium level from 120 to 135 mmol/L, the amount of Na required

= (135 mmol/L − 120 mmol/L)(0.6 × 70 L)
= (15 mmol/L)(42 L)
= 630 mmol Na

Since 1 L of NS contains 154 mmol of Na, you will require approximately 4 L of NS to raise the patient's serum level to 135 mmol/L.

b. If the patient has extracellular volume excess and edema, treat the volume excess and hyponatremia with water restriction and diuretics. Since most of these states are accompanied by secondary hyperaldosteronism, *spironolactone* is a reasonable choice of diuretic, as long as the patient is not hyperkalemic. Remember that the diuretic effect of spironolactone may be delayed for 3 to 4 days. The dose can range from 25 to 200 mg daily in adults and may be given once daily or in divided doses.

c. If the patient has a normal ECF volume, SIADH, pseudohyponatremia, or endocrine disorders should be considered.

SIADH

The diagnosis of SIADH requires that quite stringent criteria be met.

1. Hyponatremia with serum hypo-osmolality
2. Urine that is less than maximally dilute when compared with serum osmolality (i.e., a simultaneous urine osmolality that is greater than the serum osmolality).
3. Inappropriately large amounts of urine Na ($U_{Na} > 20$ mmol/L)
4. Normal renal function
5. Normal thyroid function
6. Normal adrenal function
7. Patient not on diuretics

SIADH should be treated by

1. Correcting the underlying cause or contributory factors (e.g., drugs), if present.
2. Water restriction, usually to less than insensible losses (e.g., 500 to 1000 ml/day).
3. In addition to the first two measures, patients with severe symptomatic hyponatremia (serum Na of < 115 mmol/L) may

benefit from furosemide-induced diuresis with hourly replacement of urinary sodium and potassium losses using NS. Very rarely, 3% saline will be required.

Too rapid correction of hyponatremia can result in central pontine myelinolysis and other undesirable side effects. Correct the serum sodium level *slowly*. Once the serum sodium level is greater than 120 to 125 mmol/L many of the symptoms of hyponatremia will begin to lessen.

4. *Demeclocycline* 300 to 600 mg PO BID is occasionally useful in patients with chronic symptomatic SIADH in whom water restriction has been unsuccessful.

In cases of hyperglycemia, the "true" serum sodium concentration can be estimated by the following formula:

$$\frac{(\text{observed glucose} - \text{normal glucose})\ (1.4)}{\text{normal glucose}} + \text{serum Na (observed)}$$

The factor 1.4 is an arithmetic approximation to account for the shift of water that follows glucose into the extracellular compartment, thereby "diluting" sodium.

EXAMPLE

A 35-year-old woman in diabetic ketoacidosis is admitted with the following laboratory results:

- Glucose = 83 mmol/L
- Sodium = 127 mmol/L
- Urea = 25 mmol/L
- Creatinine = 274 mmol/L

To calculate the "true serum Na," where normal glucose is taken as 5 mmol/L,

$$= \frac{(83\ \text{mmol/L} - 5\ \text{mmol/L})\ (1.4)}{5} + 127\ \text{mmol/L}$$

$$= 22\ \text{mmol/L} + 127\ \text{mmol/L}$$

$$= 149\ \text{mmol/L}$$

PSEUDOHYPONATREMIA

The diagnosis of *pseudohyponatremia* can be made by

1. Demonstrating a normal serum osmolality in the presence of hyperlipidemia or hyperproteinemia
2. Demonstrating a significant (>10 mmol/kg) osmolar gap, indicating the presence of additional osmotically active solutes, which can falsely lower the serum sodium level. This can be done by first having the laboratory *measure* serum osmolality.

You should then *calculate* serum osmolality using the following formula:

Serum osmolality (mmol/kg) =
        2 Na (mmol/L) + glucose (mmol/L) + urea (mmol/L)

If the *measured* serum osmolality is more than 10 mmol/kg greater than the calculated serum osmolality, the hyponatremia is at least partially due to the presence of osmotically active solutes, such as excess lipids or plasma proteins.

Treatment of pseudohyponatremia is restricted to correction of the underlying cause.

ENDOCRINE DISORDERS

Hypothyroidism and *Addison's disease* can be diagnosed by their typical clinical features in association with confirmatory laboratory studies. Hyonatremia in either of these two conditions responds to treatment of the underlying endocrine disorder.

ACID BASE DISORDERS

METABOLIC ACIDOSIS

- pH < 7.35
- P_{CO_2} normal or ↓
- HCO_3 ↓

The normal respiratory response to metabolic acidosis is hyperventilation with a decrease in P_{CO_2}. The expected decrease in P_{CO_2} in uncomplicated metabolic acidosis is 1 to 1.5 (ΔHCO_3).

Metabolic acidoses are conveniently divided into normal and high anion gap varieties. The normal anion gap $(Na + K) - (Cl + HCO_3) = 4$ to 12 mmol/L.

Causes

Normal Anion Gap Acidosis
Loss of HCO_3
- Diarrhea, ileus, fistula
- High output ileostomy
- RTA
- Carbonic anhydrase inhibitors

Addition of H^+
- NH_4Cl
- HCl

High Anion Gap Acidosis

- Lactic acidosis
- Ketoacidosis (IDDM, alcohol, starvation)
- Renal failure
- Drugs (aspirin, ethylene glycol, methyl alcohol, paraldehyde)
- High-flux dialysis acetate buffer
- TPN

METABOLIC ALKALOSIS

- pH > 7.45
- P_{CO_2} normal or ↑
- HCO_3 ↑

The normal respiratory response to metabolic alkalosis is hypoventilation with an increase in the P_{CO_2}. The expected increase in uncomplicated metabolic alkalosis is 0.6 (ΔHCO_3).

With Extracellular Volume Depletion and Low Urine Cl

GI losses
- Vomiting
- GI drainage (NG suction)
- Chloride-wasting diarrhea
- Villous adenoma

Renal losses
- Diuretic therapy
- Post-hypercapnea
- Non-reabsorbable anions
- Penicillin
- Carbenicillin
- Ticarcillin
- Bartter's syndrome

With Extracellular Volume Expansion and Presence of Urinary Cl

Mineralocorticoid excess
- Endogenous
    - Hyperaldosteronism
    - Cushing's syndrome
- Exogenous
    - Glucocorticoids
    - Mineralocorticoids
    - Carbenoxolone
    - Licorice excess

Alkali ingestion

Post-starvation feeding

RESPIRATORY ACIDOSIS

- pH < 7.35
- P_{CO_2} ↑
- HCO_3 normal or ↑

The normal response to respiratory acidosis is an increase in HCO_3. An immediate increase in HCO_3 occurs because the increase in P_{CO_2} results in the generation of HCO_3 according to the Law of Mass Action.

$$P_{CO_2} + H_2O \rightleftharpoons H + HCO_3$$

Later, renal tubular preservation of HCO_3 occurs to buffer the change in pH. The expected increase in HCO_3 in acute respiratory acidosis is 0.1 (Δ P_{CO_2}). The expected increase in HCO_3 in chronic respiratory acidosis is 0.4 (Δ P_{CO_2}).

Causes

CNS Depression

- Drugs (e.g., morphine)
- Lesions of the respiratory center

Neuromuscular Disorders

- Drugs (e.g., succinylcholine)
- Muscular disease
- Hypokalemia, hypophosphatemia
- Neuropathies

Respiratory Disorders

- Acute airway obstruction
- Severe parenchymal lung disease
- Pleural effusion
- Pneumothorax
- Thoracic cage limitation

RESPIRATORY ALKALOSIS

- pH > 7.45
- P_{CO_2} ↓
- HCO_3 ↓

The normal response to respiratory alkalosis is a decrease in HCO_3. An immediate decrease in HCO_3 occurs because the decrease in P_{CO_2} results in a reduction of HCO_3 according to the Law of Mass Action.

$$P_{CO_2} + H_2O \rightleftharpoons H + HCO_3$$

Later renal tubular loss of HCO_3 occurs to buffer the change in pH. The expected decrease in HCO_3 in acute respiratory alkalosis is 0.2 (Δ P_{CO_2}). The expected decrease in HCO_3 in chronic respiratory alkalosis is 0.4 (Δ P_{CO_2}).

Causes

- Physiologic conditions (pregnancy, high altitude)
- CNS disorders (anxiety, pain, fever, tumor)
- Drugs (aspirin, nicotine, progesterone)
- Pulmonary disorders (CHF, pulmonary embolism, asthma, pneumonia)
- Miscellaneous (hepatic insufficiency, hyperthyroidism)

BLOOD PRODUCTS

The maximum time over which blood products can be administered is 4 hours for 1 unit because of the danger of bacterial proliferation and RBC hemolysis. For the same reasons, if the flow rate is interrupted for more than 30 minutes, the unit must be discarded.

CONCENTRATED RBCs (PACKED CELLS)

- Volume: Approximately 300 ± 25 ml (whole blood less 200 ± 25 ml plasma; hematocrit 70 ± 5%).
- Maximum administration time: 4 hours.
- Rate of infusion: Dependent on the patient's clinical condition.
- Administration: Standard blood set for each unit hung or Y-type set if blood is to be reconstituted.
- Indications: Acute blood loss and chronic anemia if the patient is symptomatic.

De-Leukocyted RBCs

- Volume: Approximately 300 ± 25 ml.
- Maximum administration time: 4 hours.
- Rate of infusion: Dependent on the patient's clinical condition.
- Administration: Standard blood set for each unit hung plus a filter. (Filter not required if RBCs are washed.)
- Indications: Clinically significant transfusion reactions. To reduce sensitization to histocompatibility antigens.

FROZEN RBCs (DE-GLYCEROLIZED)

- Volume: Approximately 200 ml.
- Maximum administration time: 4 hours.
- Rate of infusion: Dependent on the patient's clinical condition.
- Administration: Standard blood set for each unit hung.
- Indications: Storing of rare blood groups and autotransfusion.
- *Note*: Use only in special situations.

STORED PLASMA (FORMERLY LABELLED BANKED PLASMA)

- Volume: Approximately 200 ml.
- Maximum administration time: 4 hours.

- Rate of infusion: Dependent on the patient's clinical condition.
- Administration: Standard blood set for each unit hung.
- Indications: Stable clotting factor deficiencies. Anticoagulation reversal (warfarin)
- *Note*: Supply available for immediate use.

FROZEN PLASMA (FORMERLY LABELLED FRESH FROZEN PLASMA)

- Volume: Approximately 200 ml.
- Maximum administration time: 4 hours
- Rate of infusion: Dependent on the patient's clinical condition.
- Administration: Standard blood set.
- Indications: Bleeding patients with labile coagulation factor deficiencies (Factor V or VIII).
- *Note*: Allow approximately 20 to 30 minutes to thaw.

PLATELET CONCENTRATE (RANDOM DONOR)

- Volume: Approximately 50 ml (60×10^9 platelets).
- Rate of infusion: As rapidly as possible.
- Administration: Blood components recipient set.
- Indications: Prevention or treatment of bleeding secondary to thrombocytopenia or platelet dysfunction.
- *Note*: This product is not always immediately available. The usual order is 6 to 8 units (pooled).

PLATELET CONCENTRATE (SINGLE DONOR)

- Volume: 200 to 300 ml (200 to 400×10^9 platelets).
- Maximum administration time: As per instructions from the Apheresis Unit.
- Administration: As per instructions from the Apheresis Unit.
- Indications: Patients unresponsive to random-donor platelets. Potential bone marrow recipients to limit antigen exposure.
- *Note*: Must be arranged by the patient's physician with the Apheresis Unit.

LEUKOCYTE CONCENTRATE (SINGLE DONOR)

- Volume: 200 to 300 ml (10 to 20×10^9 granulocytes).
- Maximum administration time: As per instructions from the Apheresis Unit.
- Administration: As per instructions from the Apheresis Unit.

- Indications: Administered if *all* of the following are present: (1) neutropenia $< 500 \times 10^6/L$ granulocytes, (2) fever unresponsive to appropriate 24- to 48-hour antibiotic administration, and (3) reasonable chance for survival.
- *Note*: Must be arranged by patient's physician with the Apheresis Unit.

CRYOPRECIPITATED FACTOR VIII

- Volume: 5 to 10 ml (approximately 100 units of Factor VIII and 250 mg fibrinogen per unit of cryoprecipitate).
- Rate of infusion: As rapidly as possible.
- Administration: Blood component recipient set.
- Indications: Hemophilia A, von Willebrand's disease, acquired Factor VIII deficiency, and fibrinogen replacement, e.g., DIC.
- *Note*: Dose dependent on body mass and Factor VIII level required.

FACTOR VIII CONCENTRATE

- A lyophilized, fractionated plasma product.
- Specific activity and storage conditions stated on label.
- Must be reconstituted before use.
- Indications: Moderate to severe Factor VIII deficiency and low titer of Factor VIII inhibitors.
- *Note*: Not for use in von Willebrand's disease. Consult with hematologist before administration.

FACTOR IX COMPLEX

- Lyophilized fractionated plasma product containing Factors II, VII, IX and X.
- Factor IX content and storage conditions stated on labels.
- Must be reconstituted before use.
- Indications: Factor IX deficiency. Consult with hematologist.

NORMAL SERUM ALBUMIN (HUMAN)

- Concentrates of 25% in vials of 100 ml and 5% in vials of 250 and 500 ml.
- Sodium content is approximately 145 mEq/l.
- Indications: Hypoproteinemia with peripheral edema (give 25%). Volume depletion where IV NS contraindicated (give

5%). (*Not* indicated in the asymptomatic hypoproteinemic patient.)

IMMUNE SERUM GLOBULIN

- Aqueous solution of gamma globulin in vials of 5 ml.
- For intramuscular injection.

Rh IMMUNE GLOBULIN

- Supplied in vials of 120 to 300 mcg.
- For intramuscular injection.

HEPATITIS B IMMUNE GLOBULIN (HBIG)

- Specific hyperimmune gamma globulin supplied in vials of 1 and 5 ml.
- For intramuscular injection.

BLOOD TUBES

Lavender Top (EDTA)
CBC and differential
Reticulocyte count
Direct Coombs'
G-6-PD
Sickle cell
Malaria stain
ACTH

Red/Gray ("Tiger top")
SMAC (glucose)*
Cardiac enzymes
Liver enzymes
Drug concentrations (alcohol, digoxin,
   gentamicin, and so forth)
C peptide/insulin
Protein electrophoresis
C3, C4, cryoglobulins
Osmolality
Pregnancy test

Red Top
Crossmatch
Haptoglobin
RA Latex
ANA
Tricyclic antidepressant
   concentrations

Green Top
Lactate*
Ammonia*

Blue Top (Citrate)
PT, aPTT
Fibrinogen
Circulating anticoagulants
Coagulation factor assays

Blue Top (for FDP only)
Fibrin degradation products

*These specimens must be delivered to the laboratory immediately or else put on ice for transportation.

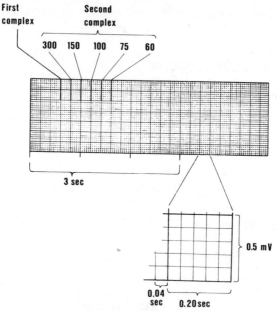

Figure A–1. Reading ECGs. Rate.

READING ECGS

RATE

Multiply the number of QRS complexes in a 6-sec period (30 large squares) (between the two large dots) by 10 = beats/min (Fig. A–1).

- Normal = 60 to 100 beats/min
- Tachycardia = > 100 beats/min
- Bradycardia = < 60 beats/min

RHYTHM

Is the rhythm regular?

Is there a P wave preceding every QRS complex? Is there a QRS complex following every P wave?

1. Yes = Sinus rhythm

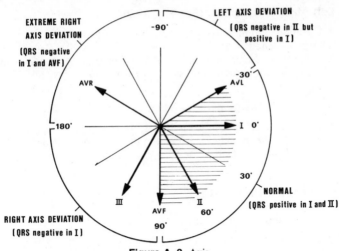

Figure A–2. Axis.

2. No P waves with irregular rhythm = Atrial fibrillation
3. No P waves with regular rhythm = Junctional rhythm. Look for retrograde P waves in all leads.

AXIS

See Figure A–2.

P WAVE CONFIGURATION

Normal P wave. Look at all leads. (See Fig. A–3a.)

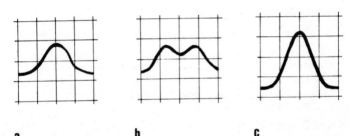

Figure A–3. Reading ECGs. P wave configuration in lead II. a = normal P wave, b = left atrial enlargement, and c = right atrial enlargement.

Left Atrial Enlargement (See Fig. A–3b.)

- Duration: 120 msec (three small squares in lead II)
  Often notched = P "mitrale"
- Amplitude: Negative terminal P wave in lead $V_1 > 1$ mm in depth *and* > 40 msec (one small square).

Right Atrial Enlargement (See Fig. A–3c.)

- Amplitude: 2.5 mm in leads II, III, or aVF (i.e., tall peaked P wave of P "pulmonale"); 1.5 mm in the initial positive deflection of the P wave in lead V_1 or V_2.

QRS CONFIGURATION

Left Ventricular Hypertrophy

1. Increased QRS voltage ("S" in V_1 or V_2 plus "R" in $V_5 > 35$ mm or "R" in aVL ≥ 11 mm.
2. Left atrial enlargement.
3. ST-segment depression and negative T wave in left lateral leads.

Right Ventricular Hypertrophy

1. "R" > "S" in V_1.
2. Right axis deviation (> + 90°).
3. ST-segment depression and negative T wave in right precordial leads.

CONDUCTION ABNORMALITIES

First Degree Block

- PR interval ≥ 0.20 sec (≥ 1 large square)

Second Degree Block

Occasional absence of QRS and T after a P of sinus origin.

1. Type I (Wenckebach's): Progressive prolongation of the PR interval before the missed QRS complex (see Fig. 12–22).
2. Type II: Absence of progressive prolongation of the PR interval before the missed QRS complex (see Fig. 12–23).

Third Degree Block

Absence of any relationship between P waves of sinus origin and QRS complexes (see Fig. 12–25).

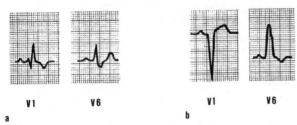

Figure A–4. Reading ECGs. QRS configuration. a = complete right bundle branch block and b = complete left bundle branch block.

Left Anterior Hemi-Block

Left axis deviation, Q in I and aVL; a small R in III, in the absence of left ventricular hypertrophy.

Left Posterior Hemi-Block

Right axis deviation, a small R in I and a small Q in III, in the absence of right ventricular hypertrophy.

Complete Right Bundle Branch Block

See Fig. A–4A.

Complete Left Bundle Branch Block

See Fig. A–4B.

Ventricular Pre-excitation

1. PR interval < 0.11 sec with widened QRS (> 0.12 sec) due to a delta wave = Wolff-Parkinson-White syndrome.
2. PR interval < 0.11 sec with a normal QRS complex = Lown-Ganong-Levine syndrome.

MYOCARDIAL INFARCTION PATTERNS

Type of Infarct	Patterns of Changes (Q waves, ST elevation or depression, T wave inversion)*
Inferior	Q in II, III, aVF
Inferoposterior	Q in II, III, aVF, and V_6
	R > S and positive T in V_1
Anteroseptal	V_1 to V_4
Anterolateral to posterolateral	V_1 to V_5; Q in I, aVL, and V_6
Posterior	R > S in V_1, positive T, and Q in V_6

*A significant Q wave is > 40 msec wide or > 1/3 rd of the QRS height. ST segment or T wave changes in the absence of significant Q waves may represent a "non-Q wave" infarct.

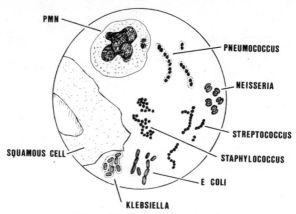

Figure A–5. Sputum Gram's stain.

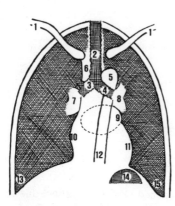

Figure A–6. Posterioanterior chest X-ray.
1. Clavicles
2. Trachea
3. Right main stem bronchus
4. Left main stem bronchus
5. Aortic knuckle
6. Superior vena cava
7. Right pulmonary artery
8. Left pulmonary artery
9. Left atrium
10. Right atrium
11. Left ventricle
12. Aortic stripe
13. Costophrenic angles
14. Gastric bubble

Figure A–7. Lateral chest X-ray.
1. Trachea
2. Left main stem bronchus
3. Right pulmonary artery
4. Left pulmonary artery
5. Aortic arch
6. Manubrium
7. Sternum
8. Breast shadow
9. Retrosternal space
10. Retrocardiac space
11. Left atrium
12. Right ventricle
13. Left ventricle
14. Inferior vena cava
15. Gastric air bubble
16. Left hemidiaphragm
17. Right hemidiaphragm
18. Costophrenic angle
19. Scapular shadows

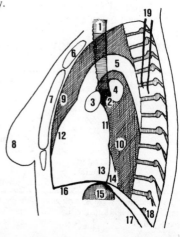

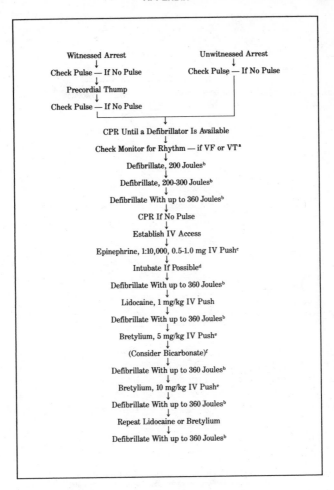

CARDIAC ARREST PROTOCOLS

Treatment Algorithm for Ventricular Fibrillation (VF) and Pulse-less Ventricular Tachycardia. The pulse and rhythm should be checked after each electric shock. If VF recurs after transient conversion, the previously successful energy level should be used for defibrillation. If intubation can be performed simultaneously with other interventions, the patient should be intubated as early in the sequence as possible; however, defibrillation and epinephrine

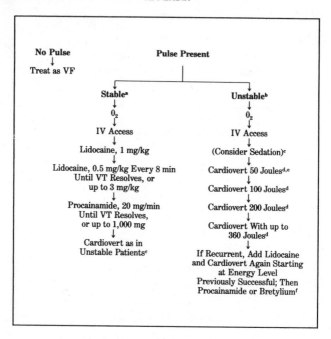

No Pulse
↓
Treat as VF

Pulse Present

Stable[a]
↓
O₂
↓
IV Access
↓
Lidocaine, 1 mg/kg
↓
Lidocaine, 0.5 mg/kg Every 8 min
Until VT Resolves, or
up to 3 mg/kg
↓
Procainamide, 20 mg/min
Until VT Resolves,
or up to 1,000 mg
↓
Cardiovert as in
Unstable Patients[c]

Unstable[b]
↓
O₂
↓
IV Access
↓
(Consider Sedation)[c]
↓
Cardiovert 50 Joules[d,e]
↓
Cardiovert 100 Joules[d]
↓
Cardiovert 200 Joules[d]
↓
Cardiovert With up to
360 Joules[d]
↓
If Recurrent, Add Lidocaine
and Cardiovert Again Starting
at Energy Level
Previously Successful; Then
Procainamide or Bretylium[f]

are more important initially if the patient can be ventilated without intubation. Epinephrine (in the indicated doses) should be administered every 5 minutes. Lidocaine hydrochloride 0.5 mg/kg every 8 minutes for a total dose of 3 mg/kg is an acceptable alternative to bretylium tosylate 5 mg/kg or 10 mg/kg. If sodium bicarbonate

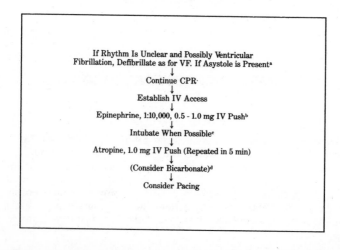

If Rhythm Is Unclear and Possibly Ventricular
Fibrillation, Defibrillate as for VF. If Asystole is Present[a]
↓
Continue CPR
↓
Establish IV Access
↓
Epinephrine, 1:10,000, 0.5 - 1.0 mg IV Push[b]
↓
Intubate When Possible[c]
↓
Atropine, 1.0 mg IV Push (Repeated in 5 min)
↓
(Consider Bicarbonate)[d]
↓
Consider Pacing

Continue CPR
↓
Establish IV Access
↓
Epinephrine, 1:10,000, 0.5 - 1.0 mg IV Push[a]
↓
Intubate When Possible[b]
↓
(Consider Bicarbonate)[c]
↓
Consider Hypovolemia,
Cardiac Tamponade,
Tension Pneumothorax,
Hypoxemia,
Acidosis,
Pulmonary Embolism

is given, a dose of 1 meq/kg followed by 0.5 mg/kg every 10 minutes may be used. (Reproduced with permission. *JAMA.* American Heart Association.)

Treatment Algorithm for Sustained Ventricular Tachycardia (VT) with Pulse. The unstable arm of the algorithm should be followed for stable patients who become unstable. Sedation before cardioversion should be considered for all patients except those with hemodynamic instability (e.g., hypotension, pulmonary edema, unconsciousness). For patients who are hemodynamically unstable, unsynchronized cardioversion is indicated to avoid delays associated with synchronization. A precordial thump may be used before cardioversion in hemodynamically stable patients. (Reproduced with permission. *JAMA.* American Heart Association.)

Treatment Algorithm for Asystole. Intubation is recommended early in the sequence if it can be accomplished simultaneously with other interventions; however, CPR and epinephrine are more important initially if the patient can be ventilated without intubation. Epinephrine should be given every 5 minutes. The endotracheal route may be used. The value of sodium bicarbonate in this sequence is unproved, and routine use is not recommended. If sodium bicarbonate is given, a dose of 1 meq/kg followed by 0.5 meq/kg every 10 minutes may be used. (Reproduced with permission. *JAMA.* American Heart Association.)

Treatment Algorithm for Electromechanical Dissociation. Intubation is recommended early in the sequence if it can be accomplished

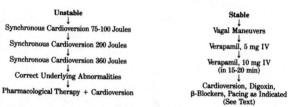

Unstable
↓
Synchronous Cardioversion 75-100 Joules
↓
Synchronous Cardioversion 200 Joules
↓
Synchronous Cardioversion 360 Joules
↓
Correct Underlying Abnormalities
↓
Pharmacological Therapy + Cardioversion

Stable
↓
Vagal Maneuvers
↓
Verapamil, 5 mg IV
↓
Verapamil, 10 mg IV
(in 15-20 min)
↓
Cardioversion, Digoxin,
β-Blockers, Pacing as Indicated
(See Text)

If conversion occurs but PSVT recurs, repeated electrical cardioversion is *not* indicated. Sedation should be used as time permits.

Paroxysmal supraventricular tachycardia (PSVT). This sequence was developed to assist in teaching how to treat a broad range of patients with sustained PSVT. Some patients may require care not specified herein. This algorithm should not be construed as prohibiting such flexibility. Flow of algorithm presumes PSVT is continuing.

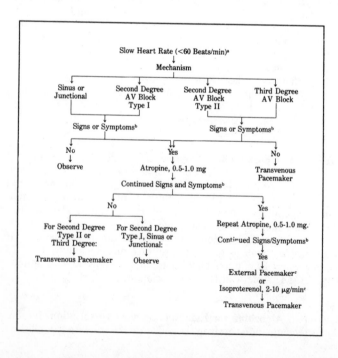

Slow Heart Rate (<60 Beats/min)[a]
↓
Mechanism

Sinus or Junctional | Second Degree AV Block Type I | Second Degree AV Block Type II | Third Degree AV Block

Signs or Symptoms[b]   Signs or Symptoms[b]

No   Yes   No
↓   ↓   ↓
Observe   Atropine, 0.5-1.0 mg   Transvenous Pacemaker

Continued Signs and Symptoms[b]

No   Yes

For Second Degree Type II or Third Degree: For Second Degree Type I, Sinus or Junctional: Repeat Atropine, 0.5-1.0 mg.
↓   ↓   ↓
Transvenous Pacemaker   Observe   Continued Signs/Symptoms[b]
                                                             ↓
                                                            Yes
                                                             ↓
                                                  External Pacemaker[c]
                                                  or
                                                  Isoproterenol, 2-10 µg/min[c]
                                                             ↓
                                                  Transvenous Pacemaker

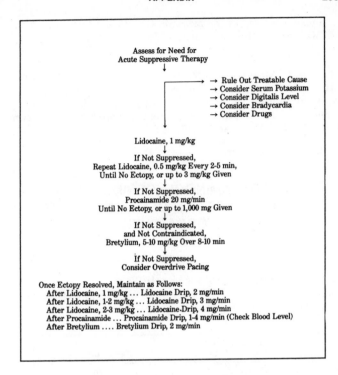

Assess for Need for
Acute Suppressive Therapy

→ Rule Out Treatable Cause
→ Consider Serum Potassium
→ Consider Digitalis Level
→ Consider Bradycardia
→ Consider Drugs

Lidocaine, 1 mg/kg

If Not Suppressed,
Repeat Lidocaine, 0.5 mg/kg Every 2-5 min,
Until No Ectopy, or up to 3 mg/kg Given

If Not Suppressed,
Procainamide 20 mg/min
Until No Ectopy, or up to 1,000 mg Given

If Not Suppressed,
and Not Contraindicated,
Bretylium, 5-10 mg/kg Over 8-10 min

If Not Suppressed,
Consider Overdrive Pacing

Once Ectopy Resolved, Maintain as Follows:
    After Lidocaine, 1 mg/kg ... Lidocaine Drip, 2 mg/min
    After Lidocaine, 1-2 mg/kg ... Lidocaine Drip, 3 mg/min
    After Lidocaine, 2-3 mg/kg ... Lidocaine Drip, 4 mg/min
    After Procainamide ... Procainamide Drip, 1-4 mg/min (Check Blood Level)
    After Bretylium .... Bretylium Drip, 2 mg/min

simultaneously with other interventions: however, epinephrine is more important initially if the patient can be ventilated without intubation. Epinephrine should be administered every 5 minutes. The value of sodium bicarbonate in this sequence is unproved, and routine use is not recommended. If sodium bicarbonate is given, a dose of 1 meq/kg followed by 0.5 meq/kg every 10 minutes may be used. (Reproduced with permission. *JAMA*. American Heart Association.)

Treatment Algorithm for Paroxysmal Supraventricular Tachycardia (PSVT). If PSVT recurs after successful cardioversion, repeated electric cardioversion is not indicated. Sedation should be used as time permits. (Reproduced with permission. *JAMA*. American Heart Association.)

Treatment Algorithm for Bradycardia. A single chest thump or cough may stimulate cardiac electrical activity and improve cardiac output; these maneuvers may be tried initially. Use of isoproterenol or an external pacemaker for patients who do not respond to atropine is a temporizing measure. (Reproduced with permission. *JAMA*. American Heart Association.)

Treatment Algorithm for Ventricular Ectopy: Acute Suppressive Therapy. If ventricular ectopy persists following correction of treatable causes, an antidysrhythmic, such as lidocaine, procainamide, or bretylium may be required. (Reproduced with permission. *JAMA*. American Heart Association.)

EMPIRIC AMINOGLYCOSIDE DOSING GUIDELINES FOR GENTAMICIN AND TOBRAMYCIN

- Loading Dose: 2.0 to 2.5 mg/kg (IBW)
- Maintenance Dose: 1.5 mg/kg (IBW) per dosing interval as suggested subsequently.

Estimated Creatinine Clearance (CrCl)	Dosing Intervals
>1.25	q8h
0.8–1.25	q12h
0.7–0.8	q16h
0.6–0.7	q18h
0.4–0.6	q24h
0.3–0.4	q30h
0.25–0.3	q36h
0.2–0.25	q48h
<0.2	Once

CALCULATION OF CrCl

$$\text{CrCl (ml/sec)} = \frac{(140 - \text{age in years}) \times 1.5}{\text{Serum creatinine } (\mu\text{mol/L})} \ (\times\ 0.85 \text{ in female})$$

CALCULATION OF THE ALVEOLAR-ARTERIAL OXYGEN GRADIENT P(A-a)O_2

The P(A-a)O_2 can be calculated easily from the ABG results. It is useful in confirming the presence of a shunt.

$$P(A-a)O_2 = PAO_2 - PaO_2$$

- PAO$_2$ = the alveolar oxygen tension calculated as shown subsequently.
- PaO$_2$ = the arterial oxygen tension measured by ABG determination.

PAO$_2$ can be calculated by the following formula:

$$PAO_2 = (PB - PH_2O) (FIO_2) - PaCO_2$$

- PB = barometric pressure (760 mmHg at sea level)
- PH$_2$O = 47 mmHg
- FIO$_2$ = the fraction of O_2 in inspired gas
- PaCO$_2$ = the arterial CO_2 tension measured by ABG determination
- R = the respiratory quotient (0.8)

Normal P(A-a)O_2 = 12 mmHg in the young adult to 20 mmHg at age 70.

In pure ventilatory failure the P(A-a)O_2 will remain 12 to 20 mmHg; in oxygenation failure it will increase.

BASIC ANTIBIOTIC SUSCEPTIBILITY GUIDELINES (SENSITIVITIES MUST BE CHECKED)*

Drug	Aerobes									Anaerobes	
++ Drug of choice **+** Effective **−** Not effective **±** Depends on sensitivity **?** Clinical efficacy not proved	Streptococcus pneumoniae, streptococci, Neisseria, Staphylococcus (penicillin sensitive)	Staphylococcus aureus (penicillin resistant)	Haemophilus influenzae	Streptococcus fecalis	Haemophilus influenzae (ampicillin resistant)	E. coli (community acquired)	Klebsiella	Pseudomonas aeruginosa	Other coliforms	Infections above the diaphragm and anaerobes excluding Bacillus fragilis	Infection below the diaphragm including B. fragilis
Amikacin	−	?	−	−	−	+	+	+	+	−	−
Ampicillin	+	−	++	++	−	++	−	−	±	+	−
Cefazolin	+	+	−	−	−	+	±	−	±	+	−

Cefotaxime	+	?	+	−	+	+	+	−	±	?	−
Cefoxitin	+	+	−	−	+	+	+	−	±	+	+
Ceftazidime	?	?	+	−	+	+	+	+	+	−	−
Cefuroxime	+	+	+	−	+	+	+	−	±	+	−
Chloramphenicol	+	+	+	+	+	+	+	−	+	+	+
Clindamycin	+	+	−	−	−	−	−	−	−	+	+
Cloxacillin/Methicillin	?	++	−	−	−	−	−	−	−	−	−
Co-trimoxazole†	±	±	+	+	+	+	?	−	−	−	−
Erythromycin	+	+	?	?	?	−	−	−	−	?	?
Gentamicin	−	?	−	−	+	+	+	+	+	−	−
Metronidazole	−	−	−	−	−	−	−	−	−	±	++
Penicillin	++	+	−	−	−	−	−	−	−	++	−
Piperacillin	+	−	+	+	+	+	+	+	+	+	+
Tetracycline	±	+	+	+	±	±	±	±	±	±	±
Tobramycin	−	?	−	−	−	+	+	++	+	−	−
Vancomycin	+	+	−	+	+	−	−	−	−	−	−

*Courtesy of St. Paul's Hospital Formulary, St. Paul's Hospital, Vancouver, British Columbia, Canada.

†Trimethoprim and sulfamethoxazole.

299

ANTIBIOTIC STANDARD DOSES FOR PATIENTS WITH NORMAL RENAL FUNCTION*

Drug	Dosage Range gm/day IV/IM (Unless Otherwise Specified)	Dosage Standard gm/dosing Interval IV/IM (Unless Otherwise Specified)	Special Comments Regarding Uses
Amikacin	15 mg/kg	7.5 mg/kg q12	For infections due to gram-negative rods resistant to gentamicin and tobramycin
Ampicillin	2–12	1 q6	
Cefazolin	3–6	1 q8	Aerobic infection with *Ps. aeruginosa*
Cefotaxime	3–12	(a) 1 q8 (b) 2 q4	(a) For susceptible bacteria resistant to less expensive agents (b) Mengingitis due to gram-negative rods resitant to ampicillin
Cefoxitin	3–8	1 q6	As a single agent in mixed infections including *B. fragilis*
Ceftazidime	3–8	1 q8	For *Ps. aeruginosa* when aminoglycosides inappropriate
Cefuroxime	2.25–4.5	0.75 q8	(a) Mixed lung infections in penicillin-allergic patients (b) *Haemophilus influenzae* resistant to ampicillin

Chloramphenicol	2–6	1 q6	Rarely indicated (irreversible aplastic anemia 1/25,000)
Clindamycin	0.6–2.4	(a) 0.6 q8 (b) 0.3 q6	(a) B. fragilis (b) Other susceptible bacteria
Cloxacillin/Methicillin	2–12	1 q6	Effective for Staph. aureus (penicillin sensitive) but penicillin is drug of choice
Co-trimoxazole†	—	—	
Erythromycin	1–4	0.5 q6	IV drug of choice for Legionella
Gentamicin	3–5 mg/kg	1.5 mg/kg q8	Initially for serious aerobic gram-negative rod infections
Metronidazole	1–2	0.5 q8	Well absorbed orally Drug of choice for Clostridium difficile pseudomembranous colitis
Penicillin	mu‡ 2–20	mu 1 q6	
Piperacillin	(a) 6–12 (b) 8–18	(a) 1.5 q4 (b) 2.0 q4	(a) For susceptible bacteria resistant to less expensive agents (b) With an aminoglycoside for leukopenic patients with Ps. aeruginosa
Tetracycline	1–2	0.5 q6	
Tobramycin	3–5 mg/kg	1.5 mg/kg q8	Better than gentamicin only for Ps. aeruginosa
Vancomycin	1–2	1 q12	For cloxacillin-resistant staphylococci

*Courtesy of St. Paul's Hospital Formulary, St. Paul's Hospital, Vancouver, British Columbia, Canada.
†Trimethoprim and sulfamethoxazole.
‡Million units.

DOSE GUIDELINES FOR THE TREATMENT OF MODERATE TO SEVERE INFECTIONS IN PATIENTS WITH VARYING DEGREES OF RENAL FUNCTION

Antibiotic	Dose	Dosing Frequency in Hours Depending on Creatinine Clearance (ml/s)			Supplement Dose for Hemodialysis
		0.8	0.8–0.4	0.4	
Acyclovir	5–10 mg/kg	8	12	24	No
Ampicillin	1–2 gm	6	6–12	12–16	Yes
Cefazolin	1–2 gm	8	12	12–14	Yes
Cefotaxime	1–2 gm	6–8	6–8	12	Yes
Cefoxitin	1–2 gm	6	8–12	12–24	Yes
Ceftazidime	1–2 gm	8	12	12	Yes
Cefuroxime	0.75–1.5 gm	8	8–12	12–14	Yes
Clindamycin	0.6 gm	8	8	8	No
Cloxacillin	0.25–1 gm	4–6	4–6	4–6	No
Gentamicin*					
Metronidazole	0.5 gm	8	8–12	12	Yes
Piperacillin	2–4 gm	4–6	6–12	12	Yes
Tobramycin*					
Vancomycin	1 gm	12			

*See page 296, Appendix.

GUIDELINES FOR DRUG THERAPY IN CARDIOPULMONARY RESUSCITATION OF ADULTS*

Drug	Indication	Dose	Frequency	Dilution	Comments
Drugs To Increase Blood Pressure or Cardiac Output					
Epinephrine hydrochloride	Degenerative rhythms (asystole, VF, bradycardia with hypotension, EMD)	0.5–1.0 mg IV, ET or 1–4 μg/min IV; titrate BP	Every 5 minutes or as needed	1 mg in 10 ml of a 1:10,000 solution	Vasopressor. Do not delay administration. Do not mix with sodium bicarbonate. Intracardiac injection is last resort. Infusion may be used. Monitor systolic and diastolic blood pressure.
Dopamine hydrochloride	Hypotension	Titrate BP, IV	Continuous infusion. Begin at 10 μg/kg/min for hypotension	Use hospital's standard dilution	Doses of 2–10 μg/kg/min have predominantly inotropic effect. Doses > 10 μg/kg/min have vasoconstrictor effect. May decrease renal, mesenteric blood flow at high doses or produce arrhythmias. Monitor ECG, BP, and organ perfusion.
Metaraminol bitartrate	Hypotension	Initial dose 5 mg IV ET; titrate BP	Continuous infusion. Begin at 5 μg/min	ET: 5 mg in 5–10 ml. IV infusions: 100 mg/250 ml D5W	May begin therapy with 5 mg (IV push or ET). Monitor BP, heart rate, urine output, organ perfusion.
Norepinephrine (levarterenol bitartrate)	Hypotension and low total peripheral resistance	Titrate BP, IV; must dilute	Continuous infusion. Begin at 1–2 μg/min	4 mg (base)/250 ml D5W	Avoid extravasation. Titrate BP. Monitor urine output and organ perfusion. (Treat extravasation with 5–10 mg phentolamine mesylate in 10–15 ml 0.9% sodium chloride injection infiltration.)
Methoxamine hydrochloride	Hypotension	Initial dose: 3–5 mg IV push; titrate BP	Continuous infusion. Begin at 5 μg/min	40 mg/250 ml D5W	May give ET. May cause bradycardia. Monitor BP, urine output, heart rate.
Phenylephrine hydrochloride	Hypotension	0.1–0.5 mg IV; titrate BP	Every 10–15 min; titrate BP	10 mg/250 ml D5W	Slow IV injection. Consider infusion.
Inotropic Agent					
Dobutamine hydrochloride	Inotropic agent (not vasoconstriction) Cardiogenic shock	Usually 2.5–10 μg/kg/min IV	Continuous infusion	250 mg/250 ml D5W	Used to improve cardiac output. May increase heart rate. Monitor BP, heart rate, organ perfusion.

Table continued on following page

303

GUIDELINES FOR DRUG THERAPY IN CARDIOPULMONARY RESUSCITATION OF ADULTS* Continued

Drug	Indication	Dose	Frequency	Dilution	Comments
Drugs to Control Heart Rhythm and Rate					
Atropine sulfate	Symptomatic bradycardia Temporary treatment of symptomatic 2nd- and 3rd-degree heart block Slow idioventricular rhythm Asystole	0.5–1.0 mg IV, ET	Every 5 minutes	Undiluted (1 mg/ 10 ml syringe)	Maximum total dose 2 mg. Doses less than 0.5 mg may cause bradycardia. May increase infarct size.
Isoproterenol hydrochloride	Hemodynamically important bradycardia unresponsive to atropine (not cardiac arrest)	Titrate heart rate, IV	Continuous infusion 0.5–10 μg/ min	1 mg/250 ml D5W	May begin therapy with small (0.2–0.5 mg) IV dose; then begin intravenous infusion. Avoid excessive heart rate, especially in acute MI. Vasodilatation with decrease in blood pressure. Alert pacer team.
Lidocaine hydrochloride	Ventricular arrhythmias. Prophylactic use in suspected MI. Follow successful cardioversion of VF. First-line drug for ventricular ectopy. VT, VF	Initial dose of 1 mg/ kg, then 0.5 mg/kg up to 3 mg/kg IV, ET	Continuous infusion (2–4 mg/ min). May repeat bolus	ET and IV push undiluted. Infusion: 1 gm/ 250 ml D5W	Give IV push over 2–3 minutes. Begin infusion when feasible. Adjust maintenance infusion based on age, weight, and cardiac and hepatic function.
Procainamide hydrochloride	Ventricular ectopy after lidocaine has failed	Loading dose of 1.0– 1.25 gm infused over 1–1.5 hours or 50 mg IV every 5 min	Continuous infusion (1–4 mg/ min)	1 g/250 ml D5W	Observe closely for cardiac depression while loading. Begin IV loading infusion at no faster than 20 mg/min. Monitor BP every 2–3 minutes until total infusion loading dose of 1–1.25 gm infused. Maintenance infusion reduced in renal failure. Monitor ECG (QRS and QT interval).
Bretylium tosylate	Resistant VF, VT (lidocaine, defibrillation, procainamide failures)	Initial dose: 5–10 mg/ kg IV. Repeat prm up to 30 mg/kg	Bolus every 15 to 30 min. Infusion 1–2 mg/ min	Undiluted for life-threatening arrhythmia. Infusion: 1 g/250 ml	Monitor for biphasic effect; Phase 1: transient hypertensive response and worsening of arrhythmia; Phase 2: antiarrhythmic effect, hypotension. Severe nausea and vomiting. Avoid in patients with increased intracranial pressure.

Drug	Indications	Dose	Rate	Dilution	Comments
Verapamil hydrochloride	Supraventricular tachyarrhythmias if carotid sinus massage unsuccessful	Initial dose: 5 mg (0.075–0.15 mg/kg) IV. Repeat dose: 10 mg	Separate first and second bolus by ≥ 10 min	Undiluted	May produce hypotension, sinus bradycardia, and A-V block. Administer with caution to patients who receive IV propranolol or who are on high doses of oral β blockers. May worsen severe heart failure.
Miscellaneous Indications					
Oxygen	Hypoxemia; all cardiopulmonary arrests	Highest possible initially; FIO2 100%	Continuous	...	Critical to improve oxygenation to the tissues.
Sodium bicarbonate	Documented metabolic acidosis. Use after defibrillation, CPR, intubation, epinephrine, antiarrhythmics fail (i.e., usually after 10 min of routine cardiac arrest sequence)	Initial dose 1 meq/kg IV; subsequent doses decrease by half	Per ABGs or every 10 to 15 min	Undiluted 44.6 meq or 50 meq in 50 mL	Must have effective ventilation. May cause hyperosmolar, hypernatremic state and impair CNS recovery. Inactivates catecholamines. Use 3-way stopcock to ease administration. Do not mix with other drugs.
Calcium salts	Only for life-threatening hyperkalemia, pre-arrest hypocalcemia, calcium blocker toxicity	10% calcium chloride: 2 ml IV Slow push	Limit use	Undiluted	Efficacy in treating asystole not proved. Avoid administration in digitalized patients. Give slowly (over at least 2 minutes IV). IV push with ECG monitoring.

*Incorporates American Heart Association and National Academy of Sciences—National Research Council 1985 national conference recommendations and the source author's experience. These guidelines should be coupled with prudent independent clinical judgment. Other drugs that may prove useful include morphine sulfate, β-blocking agents, amrinone, nitroglycerin, and sodium nitroprusside. (Reproduced with permission. Clin. Pharm. vol. 6, Feb. 1987.)
†D5W = 5% dextrose injection. EMD = electromechanical dissociation. ET = endotracheal. VT = ventricular tachycardia. VF = ventricular fibrillation. BP = blood pressure.

INDEX

Page numbers in italics indicate illustrations.
Page numbers followed by t indicate tables.